LOVE,
LOSS
&
LEADERSHIP

*Remembering in the Darkness
What I Learned in the Light*

Thea Elvin

Skrive Publications
Miramar Beach, FL
U.S.A.

Dedications

I LOVINGLY DEDICATE THIS BOOK TO JORGI, MY beautiful and unique daughter. She has wanted me to write a book for a long time. That's what daughters (or sons) do, right? Call *us* to be all we preached *they* should be from the time they could hear us from our benches of all-knowing?

Throughout my life as your mom and now through the remarkable life you have created, you've been my North Star, my reason for pushing forward, my heart. You are my greatest accomplishment. Without knowing it, you brought me out of the darkness by shining your loving light on me.

You have always told me that I am the strongest person you know. On days when I didn't feel strong or brave, your affirming words would echo in my mind. They would inspire me to go one more round in order to dig for the strong parts of my often-fractured sense of self. The strength and belief you voiced would seep into my soul, and I would find the strength to endure and to emerge as a better version of myself.

My daughter and friend, I now challenge you to take a long look in the mirror. There you will find the strongest person *I* know. With all you have been through in your young life, you have taught me more than anyone I know – most of all that pain is inevitable, but misery is optional. You have been my path back to myself. I love you with all my heart and soul.

I dedicate this book to Sofia, Gianna and Elia, my three beautiful granddaughters. Each of you is twice my child. The love that pours from you is like a soothing salve on my life. You know what I love about you? Yep! Everything!

Finally, I dedicate this book to Jonathan, my pure and kind son-in-law. Your love has broken a cycle and healed so much pain. The love you live out for your family every day is always steady and calm. If I could give you one thing in life, I would give you the ability to see yourself through my eyes, and only then would you realize how special you are to me. I love you. May God continue to bless you abundantly.

Printed in the U.S.A.

Cover design by Liz Nitardy
www.hymnsinmyheart.com

Interior formatting by Simona Meloni
www.dartfrogbooks.com

Author photograph by Jonathan Madson
www.jmadsonphotography.com

Unless otherwise noted, all scripture
verses are from the NIV Bible.
(New International Version, 2011)

ISBN 978-1-952037-16-0 (Paperback)
ISBN 978-1-952037-17-7 (eBook)

Skrive Publications
Miramar Beach, FL

www.skrivepublications.com

Contents

From the Publisher

W HEN THEA APPROACHED ME AND ASKED IF I'd be interested in helping her publish a book, I thought long and hard – for about three seconds – before saying, "Yes, of course! I'd love to help you publish your book."

I've known Thea for 25 years. Her husband Lyle was one of my best friends. My son Jonathan is married to her daughter, Jorgi. My wife and I have been friends with Thea and the rest of the Anton family for decades. When Thea told me she had been working on a manuscript, I asked to see some of what she had written. She sent me the opening chapters about losing Lyle, and I cried as I read them. When Lyle died, I missed him terribly. Not just for myself, but I missed him for my son. Can you imagine a better father-in-law for a man to have? Nope. Me either.

Anytime my wife and I had the opportunity to spend time with Lyle and Thea, we always came away better people, better spouses, better parents, better friends. That's just the way they were. They were fun, they loved each other deeply and they cared about us and our family.

Throughout the publishing journey, the same has been true. Whenever I sat down with Thea to work on her manuscript, I learned something new. She inspired me in my faith. She challenged me to think about relationships in new and different ways. She helped me become a better version of myself, a phrase she often uses.

After reviewing and revising the manuscript countless times, I went back and revisited the table of contents and noticed there was a total of 40 chapters in her book. I don't think this was an accident. Looking at the number 40 in the Bible is fascinating. It occurs no less than 146 times.

Before the great flood, it rained for 40 days and 40 nights. The Israelites wandered in the desert for 40 years before entering the Promised Land. Jesus fasted for 40 days before being tempted by the devil. The number 40 in the Bible generally symbolizes a period of hardship, trials and testing, followed, eventually, by triumph.

Love, Loss & Leadership details the hardships and trials Thea experienced, but it doesn't end there. It ends with many triumphs: the triumph of faith over fear and love over loss. The triumph of happiness over sadness and confidence over doubt. Ultimately, it will end with the triumph of life over death, both temporally and eternally.

Enjoy the book!

Dan Madson, Skrive Publications

From Me to You, Dear Reader

I N THE DEDICATION SECTION OF MY BOOK, I thanked my daughter for encouraging me to write a book. However, what I didn't mention was that I resisted the idea for many years with every fiber of my being.

I didn't feel equipped. I didn't believe in my ability to author a book. My internal voice said, "Don't be so arrogant. Everybody has a story. Who do you think you are that you could write a book and tell yours?"

I didn't know what to say or, more importantly, how to say what I wanted to say. I kept thinking, "There are a zillion books out there about grief and healing, fear and faith, love and loss, hopelessness and hope, leadership and mentoring. It's too hard. I'm not an author."

One morning, after having yet another conversation with my daughter about this, my lightning-fast mind thought to actually pray about it. I remember thinking that God would certainly agree with my thoughts on the subject thereby giving me permission to put the idea to rest and be done with it. After all, it's one thing for me to resist, but if God gave me the red light, I would have proof that I should let this foolish idea go. Uh…not so much!

I woke up at 4:37 a.m. the next morning with Psalm 81:10 going through my mind. (New International Version, 2011) "*I am the Lord your God, who brought you up out of Egypt. Open wide your mouth and I will fill it.*" What in the world? Then I read the following quote: "*Stop living in fear that you are always going to do the wrong thing. If God gives you something to do, he will anoint you to do it. Turn up the volume on your life, your voice, your dreams, your passions and yourself. You have a lot to say, so say it! Let your soul shine.*"

As time was ticking on, the end of my 41-year career was quickly approaching. Although I was still working, things were winding down on that front. I found myself going from not having enough time in the day to having very little to do. I began to feel restless and anxious.

With more time on my hands, I finally had time to write. Time to put my fingers to the keys without interruption. Time to get quiet. Time to reflect. Time to listen to God instead of just telling him what I thought I should do. This is what I know. God is God, and I am not. He will have the final word. Period.

So here I am. I started this project as a letter to a younger me, and it gradually morphed into a writing to my daughter and her three daughters.

Eventually it turned into a book. A book of thoughts and stories and lessons and ultimately, I hope, devotions about Jesus, the author and finisher of my faith.

Each day that I wrote, I found myself thinking of young women who are just starting out in life. What could I tell them that I wish I had been told?

As I wrote, I began thinking and writing more and more about God. This didn't surprise me, since he's the first one I speak to when I wake up in the morning and the last one I surrender to as I fall asleep at night.

For the record, I am not a Biblical scholar. Although I do all I can to be in the Word every day, I have never read the Bible in the order it was written. Most often, I will go to a Christian devotional book which applies to my daily life, and then go to my Bible to look up the scripture passages mentioned and meditate on them. It leads me to seek specific references, rather than simply picking up my Bible and reading randomly. If that sounds irreverent, please forgive me. The reality is I'm still learning and still growing in the Word. Day by day I'm experiencing the power it has to transform me into being more Christlike. However, at this stage of my growth, the stories about the love and grace of Jesus are most vitally important to me personally. It's through these stories that I can lean into his love and really learn about him.

You see, the Bible is my favorite book of all time, and I've read a lot of books. It's the only book that is divinely inspired and written. It was God who wrote it. Yes, the authors of the books of the Bible transcribed the words, but the Holy Spirit breathed into the minds of these writers the very words they should use. This has always astounded me, and it continues to draw me in.

Yet, to apply the principles and commands and promises with which the Bible is filled, my mind revels in books that take the Bible and bring it to the table of my heart through stories of faith, failure, forgiveness, redemption, encouragement, doubt, grace and all the rest of the stuff that we, as human beings, go through in our lives.

This is exactly what I'm praying for. That my book will bring each reader closer to the God whom I adore. Closer to Jesus, his perfect Son. Closer to the Holy Spirit, my daily Comforter.

Allow me to comment briefly about the Holy Spirit, on whom I rely every day. Synonyms in the Bible for the Holy Spirit include Comforter, Counselor, Teacher, Helper, Strengthener, Intercessor and Standby.

To me, they are more than synonyms. In my life, he has been the rock of my faith, and, honestly, a close, personal friend. He is *my* Comforter, *my* Counselor, *my* Teacher, *my* Helper, *my* Strengthener, *my* Intercessor and *my* Standby.

Oh, how I pray your relationship with the Holy Spirit will be as fulfilling as mine!

As I've grown older, the love for my Savior has become purer and more childlike. For now, my desire is that I can put down on paper some of the things I wish someone would have told me when I was growing up, thereby weaving them into a tapestry of stories that will bless your life.

Do you ever wonder if a younger you would listen to the guidance that you now want to give to those you love? I sure do.

I'm sure a lot of the early wisdom I longed for as a young woman would have fallen on deaf ears. Still, those ideas would have been there, marinating in my subconscious mind until all the flavors began to meld together. Until a wholeness of life began to emerge enough for me to be a blessing to someone else, despite my stubbornness.

My deepest prayer is that my words will in some way speak to anyone else who has lived or is living in the dark. I pray as I write that my words will guide you to the light of God's staggering love. I pray that my words will not only bless you but honor the one who continues to carry me, catch me, love me, forgive me, expect more from me, want more for me and is gracious to me when I don't always live out the faith I proclaim to have. This grace, God's underserved love for me, is one of the fundamental, most important truths in the Bible. As I lean into him, he always holds me.

I pray that the Holy Spirit will be with you as you read. I pray that God's grace will cover your life. Finally, I pray that the words on these pages and the meditation of my heart will be pleasing to you, O Lord.

And so, in remembering the lessons I learned in the darkness, I continue in the light.

With love, Thea

Into the Darkness

1

Grief

"The darker the night, the brighter the stars; the deeper the grief, the closer to God!" ~Fyodor Dostoevesky

MARCH 9, 2013, WAS THE LONGEST DAY OF my life. My guy (as I called him) had been battling lung cancer for 17 months. His name was Lyle, but I called him L, honey or baby.

I'm going to talk about him a lot. He's worthy of mention. From his initial diagnosis to the moment he took his last breath, he was joyful. Was he happy he was going through this? No. Did he have indescribable suffering at times? Yes. But happiness is altogether different than joy. Happiness is dependent upon circumstances. Joy is a choice. For a Christian, joy is one of the fruits of the Spirit. Lyle chose joy.

When starting chemotherapy, Lyle would say things to me like, "Ain't nothin' to it but to do it, baby." He would also say things like, "We're all terminal, T." Once, near the end of his life, I was sitting on the side of the tub talking to him as he was taking a bath. He was wearing the cross he wore every day.

I said, "Do you want to take the cross with you?"

He smiled and said, "No, T. I'm going to the man who made the cross." He never felt sorry for himself. He never asked, "Why me?" Never. Not once.

My eyes filled with tears and I said to him, "You've taught me how to live; now you're teaching me how to die?" He just smiled and winked.

In the end, hospice was Lyle's choice, as his desire was to die at home.

And so, on March 9, 2013, our family room was filled with family members. It occurred to me that this might be why it's called a family room. Gathering is a common occurrence when someone in our traditional Greek family is dying. All who can come together to say goodbye, do so.

What I didn't expect was for our family room to also be filled with angels.

From the time she was a little girl, my daughter, Jorgi, has seen angels. We would be in church and she would lean over to me and ask, "Mama, do you see them?"

I would say, "Where?"

She would point to a location in the church with urgency as if to say, "Don't you see them?"

I would just shake my head no. I wish I could have seen them, but I never did.

That day in our family room, she was no longer a little girl. She was turning 30 the next day. I looked at her and her eyes were filled with tears. I assumed it was because her dad was dying in the bedroom next to us. I asked her if she was okay. She said, "Mom, this entire room is filled with angels." She said, "It's not scary, but it is overwhelming." Once again, I didn't see them, but she absolutely did.

The hospice nurses had told me there were specific physical things that would happen when someone was ready to die. That time had come. Although Lyle had been in a coma for a couple of days, I was allowing other people to be in the bedroom with him to say their goodbyes. During such times, I would wait in the family room. My sister Nia came from the bedroom and told me that Lyle was doing something odd with his mouth. That was one of the signs. I ran in, put my arms around him, told him how much I loved him and purposely put my fingers on the pulse of his wrist. Just a few moments later, he took his last breath and my fingers felt his pulse go still. I started to weep, fell to my knees and said, "Praise God." I was praising God that his suffering was over. I was praising God for the beautiful man whose body was in my arms, but whose spirit was with the Lord. I was praising God because it was all I knew how to do.

I looked up and all the family members who had been

in the family room were now in the bedroom with us. They were all crying. Love does that.

According to Jorgi, the angels had moved to the bedroom too.

Ultimately, we all stood together in the bedroom as the people from the mortuary came to get Lyle's body. They put him in a body bag and then wrapped him in the American flag. Together, with tear-stained faces, our family saluted Lyle. He had served in the United States Air Force, but this isn't why we saluted. We saluted his life and his influence. We saluted his love and his friendship. We were wishing him a beautiful journey home.

My daughter told me that the moment Lyle died, the angels were gone. There was no doubt in my mind they were escorting him into heaven. *"And the angels carried him to Abraham's side." Luke 16:22*

They rolled Lyle out into the darkness and placed him in their waiting vehicle to take him to the mortuary. I remember that we all followed them out. We had a detached garage that was also Lyle's workshop where he constantly had music playing. As we passed by the open door, the music was on. It was loud, and it was awesome. Exactly how he would have wanted it. I can't remember what was playing, but it was probably Dean Martin, Huey Lewis and the News or Human Nature. Everyone smiled and kept walking toward the front of the house where the car was waiting. As they tried to put Lyle in the back, the gurney kept getting stuck and would not quite go in. Out of sheer instinct I said, "That a boy, L!" Everyone started laughing through their tears. They finally managed to get him inside the car and as they drove away, we all held on to each other and walked back into the house. The house whose nooks and crannies had been filled to the brim with love that anyone entering could feel it. The house that would never again feel like home to me. Not without my guy.

I went into the bedroom and fell on the bed and wept so hard I couldn't catch my breath. I could feel someone standing next to me and rubbing my back. I thought it was my daughter, but I couldn't even look up. After what seemed like an eternity, I looked up and saw it was my 87-year-old mom. This shook me up. For her to have to watch me like this, her own child so heartbroken, was sad beyond measure.

I tried to pull myself together. I tried for a very long time, but grief caught up with me. The beautiful life I knew with Lyle was over. My journey into the darkness had begun.

It may sound morbid, but when Lyle slipped into a coma, I went online and began to read about the process of dying. I wanted to know exactly what a person typically goes through after suffering with a long illness.

I discovered that Lyle had been through many of the things described, but there were more to come that I believed would be difficult to bear watching. Lyle was a humble man, but he had a strong sense of dignity. I felt such a strong pull in my spirit to spare him losing that, even in death.

I called Lyle's sister, my dear friend Janny. I asked her to reach out to her church members to see if there was a specific prayer that we could pray to ask God to allow Lyle to bypass the final steps of suffering. She did and got back to me within a couple of hours.

With Lyle lying on his hospice bed, Janny and I went into our walk-in closet, held hands, bowed our heads and she prayed this prayer:

"Lord, your Word says that whenever two or more are gathered in your name, you are there in the midst of them. We thank you for your Spirit who is with us and for hearing us as we pray for Lyle. We love him and we know you love him even more. We know what the books say about the process of dying, but we ask you now, Father, to lift the final parts of suffering from Lyle and take him home without having him go through them. In your precious name we pray, Amen."

Lyle never went through the final steps of suffering. He simply didn't suffer them. He passed into heaven with his dignity and honor in place.

No one can ever convince me that God is not gracious. Ever.

Dear Heavenly Father,

Thank you for Lyle's life, for the way he loved and for the profound influence he had. Thank you for the way he loved you and the stand he took for you without hesitation. Thank you for his bravery, not only in life, but as he went through the valley of the shadow of death. He is yours. You have called him by name. Heaven will be much more fun now. I know he's having a ball!

In Jesus' name, Amen.

FOR YOUR OWN READING: JOHN 11

2
I Can't Sleep

"Sleep doesn't help if it's your soul that's tired." ~Anonymous

IT STARTED THE EVENING THEY TOOK LYLE'S body away. I couldn't sleep. I tossed and turned and cried and cried. Still, I couldn't sleep. Finally, completely exhausted and drained, I took an over-the-counter sleep aid. Can't remember which one. I was scared to take it, as I had never taken one before. But exhaustion won out and I took it. I fell asleep and during that sleep, I was finally able to forget that my world was different, seemingly broken and sad.

I opened my eyes and life was going on all around me. Some family members were planting ivy in my front yard, knowing I'd wanted it there for a long time. It was a beautiful gesture of love and support. I looked through my bedroom window and watched them working. I was so touched that I began to cry again. This time from seeing this wonderful act of kindness.

Finally it dawned on me. I wasn't the only one grieving Lyle's death. However, self-absorption was slowly becoming my constant companion. It was like an unconscious default to the grief that had drained me during the months leading up to Lyle's death. In retrospect, I can now see that while I was trying to survive emotionally, I seldom stopped to think about how others were also grieving. Numbness not only blinded me to my own feelings, but also blinded me to the feelings of those around me. In a perfect world, I would have (and should have) been more aware of the feelings that others were having. Sadly, I was fighting so hard to stay level myself that I lost my natural feelings of empathy. It wasn't until much later, when the numbness began to thaw, that I could see things from the perspective of others who loved Lyle so much.

"Forgive yourself for not knowing what you didn't know before you learned it."
~Anonymous

When it came time to sell Lyle's truck, Putt, my brother-in-law, helped me with the process. Actually, he sold it for me. When time came for the buyers to pick it up at my home, Putt was there with me to make sure all went according to plan. It gave me confidence to have him there with me. It wasn't until the buyers drove Lyle's truck around the corner of our street and out of view, that I realized just how much Putt was grieving. As I put my arms around his waist, and leaned on him, I started crying. He hugged me, and tears began to fall down his cheeks. "I'm sorry, Putt," I said.

He said, "T, I'm not crying for you. I'm crying for me. I miss him every day."

I've learned that we can only connect our dots backward, not forward. As Maya Angelou once wrote, "Do the best you can until you know better, then when you know better, do better."

Yes, ma'am, and Amen!

Dear Lord,

Thank you for your love that is so strong it outlasts loss or grief. Thank you for Lyle's friends and family and the love they had for each other. Thank you for making me aware of others' sorrow amid my own and for restoring my sense of empathy. Bless those who bless me through their feelings and actions, even while bearing their own grief.

In Jesus' name, Amen.

"Lord grant me the ability to forgive
myself for past stumbles and falls,
to correct what I can, and accept
what I can't, and the courage to
try again, this time a bit wiser."
~Anonymous

FOR YOUR OWN READING: 2 CORINTHIANS 1

3
Got a Lump in Your Throat?

"All the art of living lies in the fine mingling of letting go and holding on."
~Havelock Ellis

BEFORE I EVEN OPENED MY EYES, I COULD feel a lump in my throat and a sense of foreboding surrounding me like a heavy fog. I turned my thoughts to Jesus and prayed that he would lift this feeling from me. I asked the Holy Spirit to fill me with his love, so that fear would have no place in me.

I shook off grief as a daily assignment, yet, at times its fragments clung to me with all their might.

I used to question how I could know and believe the

"I call on the Lord in my distress, and he answers me."
~Psalm 120:1

Scriptures when feelings of doubt and despair washed over me like waves. It caused me to breathe deeply in order to just breathe normally again.

I repeated my friend Kathy's mantra over and over. It has now become mine. *God is in me, God is with me, God is for me.*

While I remembered to go to the Word of God for refuge, I recalled the words of the great George Mueller: *"The beginning of anxiety is the end of faith, and the beginning of true faith is the end of anxiety."*

As I surrendered it all, even for a moment, I could begin another day believing in his promises, my feelings notwithstanding, and live out each day basking in his healing and covered by his grace.

Healing takes time, and I was keenly aware that I had to surrender myself to the emptiness I still felt, since the one that I loved with all my heart and soul was no longer there. *God is in me, God is with me, God is for me.*

Dear Lord,

In my distress I cry out to you. You hear my prayers and answer them. Thank you for the peace you deliver to my soul and for the healing words that I need each day. You are my strength and my helper whenever I am in need.

I ask for your blessing on my life this day.
In Jesus' name, Amen.

"I am the Lord who heals
you." ~Exodus 15:26

FOR YOUR OWN READING: JOHN 16

4
A Widow

"Days are not the way they were when he was alive." ~Christine Thiele

I'LL NEVER FORGET STANDING AT THE RECEP-tionist's desk outside the oncologist's office and hearing the receptionist say to me, "Marital status?"

I said, "Excuse me?"

She said, "You didn't fill out the section on the form that asks your marital status."

I said, "Oh." And then I thought, "Did someone just kick me in the stomach?"

Again, without looking up she said, "Marital status?"

I said "Oh." I paused and then said, "Widow." She checked that box without looking up.

When this happened, it had been nearly seven years since my husband died. My beautiful, uncommonly handsome, kind, funny, brave, emotionally and physically strong, loving husband died. I know people might tell me not to say this, but I'm saying it anyway. My life has never been the same. On occasion, the grief I felt at 5:55 p.m. on March 9, 2013, while holding Lyle as he took his last breath, is still like a raw wound. It's still as physically, emotionally and mentally profound as it was in that very moment. I miss everything about him, and I miss the woman I was when I was with him. I look around at other widows and they seem to have moved on. This, of course, is simply my interpretation based on how things look, not on real knowledge. Many widows that I know have remarried or are dating regularly. Others have thrown themselves into their work and are making a remarkable difference.

> "Blessed are those who mourn, for they will be comforted."
> ~Matthew 5:4

I actually remember someone saying to me right after Lyle died, "Oh man! I can only imagine all the amazing things you're going to do in your career now that you'll have so much time on your hands!" Nothing could have been further from the truth.

So, the questions began. What's wrong with me? Why can't I suck it up? What am I doing?

They say that work is the antidote for grief, but, seriously, I felt like a woman wearing a pair of brown shoes in a room full of tuxedos.

As a Christian, I have no doubt that Lyle is in heaven. He had a simple yet convicted faith in Jesus as his Savior. He didn't talk about it unless he was asked about it, but he lived it. He was a man's man with a tender heart and an incredible sense of self. I would often say, "From Yale to jail, he would be the same person." He was one of the purest people I've ever known.

I only heard him say things that could be perceived as negative about three people in all the time I knew him. Because I agreed with his opinion of each of the three, I understood his need to say them. He didn't belabor the points. He said them and moved on. He was like that with everything. He didn't have time for grudges. He was a fireman who loved his work. He used to say he whistled all the way to work and all the way home for 28 years. Yet, he never brought his work home with him.

The stories I heard about the heroic things he did or the horrific things he went through on the job never came from him. They came from the other firefighters who loved and respected him so much. He only shared the funny stuff. He retired 10 years before he died. I'm extraordinarily grateful for our 20 years of marriage, but those 10 years were an extra, cherry-on-top blessing for both of us.

He was tough and tender. His friends called him MacGyver because he could fix anything. I used to say that he could go into the dessert with a rubber band and come out with a boat.

He would cry every time he prayed, whether it was before a meal with family or just the two of us. Every time. He loved God. He lived with no regrets, and he knew that he was a forgiven sinner. He lived with absolute conviction that he was forgiven the moment he asked for forgiveness. Unlike me, I don't think he ever took the same sin to the foot of the cross twice. He knew he was human, and that God sent Christ to save him, because he couldn't save himself. He lived his life accordingly. That's why he could fall asleep anywhere.

True story. When we were first dating, we were sitting on the floor in front of the couch watching TV. My back was leaning against the couch, and he was lying in front of me with his head in my lap. I started to scratch his head. I'm not exaggerating. Five seconds after I started scratching his scalp, he was not only sound asleep, but snoring. Out of sheer disbelief, I woke him up by gently nudging him. I said "Honey, you fell asleep!"

He said, "Yeah. I was dreaming that I was mowing my grandpa's lawn."

What? Man, that was awesome! "There's no pillow as soft as a clear conscience," I thought. That was my guy. Leave it at the cross. Don't pick it back up. Do better next time. Simple. Pure. I didn't get that gene.

I once read that a happy marriage is a union of two good forgivers. Amen to that! I have also learned that the one with the highest self-esteem will be the first to take a step toward healing. That was my guy, and his example took me to a higher level of forgiveness. He was always willing to be the first to say, "I'm sorry." Even if he didn't know what he was sorry for. (Women do that to men, don't we?) He taught me that it's more important to be happy than to be right.

I once heard a comedian tell this story. He said, "I wake up in the morning next to my wife and the first thing I say is, 'I'm sorry.'"

She says, "For what?"

He said, "I don't know, I just wanted to get it over with."

I will never forget our first heated disagreement. Of course, I can't remember what we were disagreeing about, but it started to get heated. We began to raise our voices and started talking over each other. Suddenly we stopped and just looked at each other, knowing this was going nowhere fast. I turned around and started to stomp away. (Isn't that a lovely picture? Uh, not so much.)

> "He heals the brokenhearted and binds up their wounds."
> ~ Psalm 147:3

Before I could take ten steps, I heard Lyle whistling. Whistling? What? Yep. I whipped around and saw him happily walking away, still whistling.

I said, "L!"

He turned around and said, "Yeah?"

I said, "Were you just whistling?"

He said, "Yeah, why?"

I said, "Because we were just in a huge argument not more than five seconds ago!"

He said, "T, let me tell you something. If you ever leave me, I'm goin' with ya, so there's no reason not to whistle."

I learned right there that I could disagree with him and he with me, but no one was ever going anywhere. That funny incident solidified our foundation of complete trust, coupled with the rare certainty that we could each be authentically unique and still be loved unconditionally. It gave me the confidence to speak my mind. Although our discussions sometimes became heated, I must emphasize that they were *always* respectful. It was safe for both of us to be uncompromisingly honest and open. Our love was unconditional. Rare. Pure. Safe.

Lyle was the love of my life. He was my best friend, my companion, my helper, my lover and my teacher. He helped me to lighten up. He made me laugh until my stomach ached. He made me feel safe and he loved me deeply every single day. That's why I have a lump in my throat. That's why tears still welled up in my eyes as I wrote this seven years after he died.

Dear Lord,

Thank you for your liberating love for me and all mankind. Thank you for 20 beautiful years of marriage to one of the all-time great men. Thank you for gifting him with high self-esteem and an unselfish love toward me. Thank you for your promises of heaven. I can't even begin to imagine how happy Lyle is there, but your Word gives me a glimpse. You know my longing for him, yet I thank you that day by day you are healing my heart by filling it with your Holy Spirit.

In Jesus' name, Amen.

"In peace I will lie down and sleep, for you alone, Lord, make me dwell in safety." ~Psalm 4:8

FOR YOUR OWN READING: 1 THESSALONIANS 4

5
Change

"People change and forget to tell each other." ~Anonymous

PRIOR TO MY RETIREMENT, I WORKED IN THE same career for 41 years. I was extraordinarily blessed to do something that I loved for most of my adult life. I'm keenly aware of how rare this is. Not the length of service but the 'loving what you do' part. I've heard it said that people can spend 41 years climbing the ladder of success, only to one day realize it was leaning against the wrong wall. I'm grateful that this has not been the case for me.

Then, one day after Lyle passed away, the things that I had always looked forward to felt like a burden. Worse, I felt guilty for feeling that way. After all, I considered myself to be the Grand Poohbah of positive attitudes. I actually taught the importance of having that attitude throughout my entire career. One of my all-time favorite quotes is from Zig Ziglar. He said, "I'm so positive, I'd go after Moby Dick in a rowboat and take the tartar sauce with me." I mean, that's being positive, right?

So, I didn't talk about feeling burdened, and I pushed through. Discipline always guided those motions. However, the dread I felt on a day-to-day basis was so strong that I knew I couldn't have done it through sheer discipline alone. Looking back and even at the time, I knew that it was my deep faith in God and my sense of responsibility that carried me through. Day by day. Hour by hour. Sometimes, minute by minute.

I've heard it said that grief is the price we pay for love. I get that. The love that Lyle and I shared has been worth every moment of grief.

"And hope does not put us to shame, because God's love has been poured out into our hearts through the Holy Spirit, who has been given to us."
~Romans 5:5

The side effects of grief, however, can be brutal, unexpected and frightening.

In his book *A Grief Observed*, C.S. Lewis wrote about the feelings associated with the death of his wife: *"No one ever told me that grief felt so like fear. I am not afraid, but the sensation is like being afraid. The same fluttering in the stomach, the same restlessness, the yawning. I keep on swallowing. At other times it feels like being mildly drunk, or concussed. There is a sort of invisible blanket between the world and me. I find it hard to take in what anyone says. Or, perhaps hard to want to take it in. It is so uninteresting. Yet I want the others to be about me. I dread the moments when the house is empty. If only they would talk to one another and not to me."*

I can't begin to express the great comfort it gave me as I read his words. To know that such a man of faith felt the same way I felt, admitted it and wrote about it. I took a long deep breath when I read his words and I actually exhaled.

I still wonder if that feeling of fear ever left him? I'll ask him when I get to heaven.

I read that when a plant lives in a dry and barren climate, its roots drive deeper and deeper into the soil to get the water it needs. This forces the plant to develop a root system that is far beyond any normal plant because it's forced to go deeper to be nourished. Looking back, I can now see that during my dry and barren seasons, I was forced to go deeper into the grace of God's love to build a stronger foundation of faith. *"Therefore we do not lose heart. Though outwardly we are wasting away, yet inwardly we are being renewed day by day. For our light and momentary troubles are achieving for us an eternal glory that far outweighs them all. So we fix our eyes not on what is seen, but on what is unseen, since what is seen is temporary, but what is unseen is eternal." 2 Corinthians 4:16-18* These seasons have accomplished in me what may never have been accomplished any other way. Each day I still ask the Lord for the grace to surrender. I trust that he will pour his grace out on me in the desert times of my life. I know that he will help me persevere for my own well-being and for his glory.

Dear Lord,

On the days that I wake up remembering that Lyle isn't here, I know the ache that I feel can be framed by your love and your purpose. For that I thank you. I ask you, Lord, to continue to lift fear from me, for I know it doesn't come from you. Cover me, I pray, with your white light of protection. Lyle is with you. I am still here. Bless me, Lord, so that I may be a blessing to all I meet today.

In Christ's name, Amen.

FOR YOUR OWN READING: ISAIAH 41

6

Complicated Grief

"God gave us memory so that we might
have roses in December." ~J.M. Barrie

AS I MENTIONED EARLIER, THERE WERE TIMES
when I didn't enjoy my work but did it anyway. What
I didn't mention was that during those times, I was
doing it feeling completely numb. In that numbness, I
was unknowingly putting myself into a vulnerable state.
Vulnerable to the opinions of others, some of whom at
other times in my life, I would never have listened to nor
taken advice from.

Despite having what I (and others) considered to be a
dream career, the circumstances of my life had blinded me to
the point that I didn't even recognize how I'd been knocked
to my knees physically, mentally and emotionally.

These were the times when I realized how ill-equipped
I was to handle things with personal grace and my own
grit and strength. Prior to those difficult, emotional events,

I thought I had everything I needed in my life's toolbelt to handle anything. Looking back, I now understand clearly that the emotion of grief took me to some very dark places.

After Lyle's passing, I went to two grief counselors, both lovely and kind. Neither mentioned the phrase 'complicated grief' to me. Or maybe they did, and I didn't hear it. It's possible, if not probable.

Nevertheless, it was on a podcast where I first heard the concept of complicated grief. It described in detail exactly what I had been going through. Loss of spouse, yes, but also the loss of everything associated with him: emotional and mental support, financial security, relationships, a feeling of safety, a helper. The list goes on. To heal from it, you must grieve all of it. "Such a special treat!" said no one ever.

There was a staggering shift that darkness caused which seemed to overwhelm my soul. It was only through a willingness to acknowledge it and a genuine fight to move back into the light that the sunshine of my soul could be restored. *"For you were once darkness, but now you are light in the Lord. Live as children of light." Ephesians 5:8*

It was frightening for me to open myself up again. To some degree it still is. It was difficult to stop the intentional isolation, which on some delusional level I believed was protecting me. It was necessary, I now realize, to allow myself to be vulnerable to pain again.

I remember the year my husband died, I went to get a massage. After the massage the therapist, a woman I'd never met before, asked me whom I had lost. I was stunned by her question. In a split second the trigger was pulled and the lump in my throat appeared. Tears welled up in my eyes. "My husband," I said, "but how did you know I lost someone?"

She said, "You walked in here protecting your heart. Your posture, the way you walked in slumped over, the way you covered your heart with your arms and hands, it was obvious to me that you were trying to protect yourself from pain. You don't know me, but I'm suggesting that you stand up straight again, and physically open your posture to expose your heart to the world. Eventually, you will learn to live and laugh again. Wouldn't he have wanted that?"

"Ouch," I thought, "and Amen!" It was such an intuitive and helpful comment.

I never even asked for her name. She was a blessing sent to me by God. God knows her name. I'll just call her Angel.

I had no idea I was slumped over. Me? I don't slump! As a matter of fact, when I was growing up, if my proud Greek father ever saw me walking with my head down, he would take his hand, quickly and not always gently, lift my chin and say, "Lift your head up! You're an Anton. Walk proud." I didn't appreciate it at the time, but it stuck with me. So, for her to say I was slumping. What? No way!

And covering my heart? I had no clue. How could I be covering my heart? Hesitantly, I pulled my shoulders back and stood up straight. I put my hands out to the sides of me and put my chest out as far as it could go. (I've always been flat-chested, so that took some doing.) I took a deep breath, and I began to weep.

It was the beginning of my way back to me. It would take a while, a long while, but it was the beginning.

I think it was Dr. Phil McGraw who said, "You can't change what you don't acknowledge." Acknowledged. I became willing to open myself up, and that willingness, for me, was monumental.

The willing? Destiny guides them. The unwilling? Destiny drags them. I didn't want to be dragged anywhere. With my head up and the promise that the Lord himself would go before me and never leave me, I took one more step toward the light, fears and all. *"The Lord himself goes before you and will be with you; he will never leave you nor forsake you. Do not be afraid; do not be discouraged." Deuteronomy 31:8*

Heavenly Father,

Thank you, Lord, for the stranger you placed in my life. Thank you for allowing her to awaken the scared little girl who had been walking around this world with an invisible sign that said, "Stay away from me." I still wear that sign at times, but by your grace, it's getting easier to shed. Thank you for your promise to go before me. I can move forward remembering that you're already there.

In Jesus' name, Amen.

FOR YOUR OWN READING: EPHESIANS 5

7

Who Me? Yes You! Couldn't Be! Then Who?

"Life is what happens to us while we're making other plans." ~John Lennon

IT WAS A BIG, HEAVY PLASTIC GARBAGE CAN lid, the kind you see covering the garbage cans in a neighborhood where everyone takes their garbage out on Tuesdays. You know the ones I mean? Anyway, it was big and heavy. I am small and light. It fell on me one day as I was trying to close it and slammed down on my left breast. I instinctively rubbed the area that was hit, trying to take the sting away. As I did, I felt a lump.

After losing Lyle to cancer, and with my sister right in the middle of treatments for cancer herself, this little lump didn't set well with my Inner Knower, another name I have for the Holy Spirit. I went to the doctor, who, to rule things out, sent me to a surgeon. The surgeon felt it and told me that he thought it was a hematoma from the garbage can lid slamming down on me. "Nothing to worry about," he said.

Relieved, I moved along, until I went to see a new gynecologist for an initial appointment to establish a relationship. She did a breast exam, felt the lump and sent me right back to that surgeon. This time, because the hematoma hadn't gone away, he sent me to get a breast biopsy. (Ya think?)

A few days later, I was back in the surgeon's office sitting on this table in the middle of a cold room, wearing a not-so-cool looking hospital gown, talking to a nurse who was very rigid. She wouldn't even look me in the eye as she took my blood pressure, temperature and weight. My Inner Knower was on full alert as I watched her. I think she missed school the day they taught the lesson called *How to Have a Warm and Reassuring Bedside Manner.* "The doctor will be in shortly," she said as she walked out.

I just sat there. As much as I tried to stay positive, I could feel the burning in my eyes as I did all I could to hold back tears as they fought for their rightful spot.

I remember swallowing a lot. This helped keep my emotions at bay. I did deep breathing, like in a yoga class. I calmed myself down as I waited for the doctor to come. "He'll be in shortly," the nurse had said. Shortly? Who made that up? He'll be in shortly is like when you're a little kid and you have a loose tooth that's dangling and your parent says, "Oh, honey, it's okay, it'll come out shortly." Well, it didn't. As a little kid it seemed to take forever when you were waiting for the money from the tooth fairy and your tooth just kept hanging there. Forever!

That's how I felt. He was taking forever. The good part in the waiting was that my lightning-fast mind remembered to pray. I don't remember exactly what I prayed for, only that I thanked God that he was with me and that he would never leave me. I think the verse from Romans 8:26 summed up my feeble attempt to find the words to pray. "*In the same way, the Spirit helps us in our weakness. We do not know what we ought to pray for, but the Spirit himself intercedes for us through wordless groans.*"

Yep. Groans – inaudible to the naked ear, mind you – but that's what I was sitting there doing. Praying with groans too deep for words.

Finally, the doctor came into the cold room and in a straight-forward manner said, "You have breast cancer. You caught it early. From the biopsy, I believe that it's Stage 1. I've set up an appointment for you to see an oncologist right away."

You could have given me a glass of my favorite wine or a piece of my mom's incomparable fried chicken along with that statement, and I *still* couldn't have swallowed it.

There was a rhyme that we used to say when we were kids. We'd say, "Who stole the cookie from the cookie jar?"

Then we'd shout a name of one of the kids playing with us, "Susie stole the cookie from the cookie jar!"

Then Susie would say, "Who me?"

In unison the rest of the kids would shout, "Yes, you!"

And Susie would say, "Couldn't be!"

Together we'd shout, "Then who?" Then we'd start the game all over again with another kid's name being shouted as the stealer of the cookie from the cookie jar.

This was no rhyme, no game, and this wasn't about a cookie, but that's how I felt. Who, me? Absolutely could *not* be. To my knowledge, aside from my sister who was being treated for lung cancer from smoking since she was a teenager, and my paternal grandfather who had throat cancer from the same thing, no one in my biological family had suffered from cancer. It just wasn't something I thought I'd ever get.

Who me? Yes, you! It was a bitter pill to swallow.

The doctor said some things to me about the type of cancer it was, the stage it was at and what the treatment plan would be. "Waa, waa, waa," was all I heard, like Lucy in the Peanuts cartoon. I was numb and scared, so I called my daughter at work.

I can't remember exactly what I said to her, except that I needed her to be with me. She asked me what was wrong.

I told her that I just found out that I had breast cancer. She said nothing except, "I'll be there as fast as I can." She got coverage, left work and came directly to the cold waiting room where I was still sitting in shock. She said, "Mom, you're going to beat this and I'm going to be right by your side the entire time!" To her credit, she kept her word.

This happened in 2014. I got three different opinions. All three oncologists confirmed that I had Stage 1 breast cancer. Based on the type of cancer it was, they all suggested chemotherapy and radiation treatments. The first oncologist I saw was the one who treated my husband. With all the respect and verbal skills I could muster, I thanked her and politely told her that I preferred to see someone else. I assured her it had nothing to do with her abilities or my belief in her. She was a wonderful doctor and was very good to Lyle. I told her that I just didn't want to relive going to her office and being reminded of the 17 months of appointments I had been through. She assured me this was fine, gave me another recommendation and I went there.

In the meantime, I had heard of another oncologist who was highly rated and recommended. I went to see her, and I loved her from the moment I walked in. We talked and she said something to me that gave me the strength to face the future with confidence. She simply said, "Thea, you're going to be just fine." I felt like I could climb the highest mountain in the world when she said that. My fear turned to hope. Turns out that my insurance didn't cover her. That was okay. "You're going to be just fine" was a gift of words that God gave to me through her that day, and they sustained me through-out chemotherapy, the side effects of it, losing my hair and radiation treatments. *"The tongue has the power of life and death, and those who love it will eat its fruit." Proverbs 18:21*

This doctor spoke life over me in one sentence. We can't choose a diagnosis once it's been given, but we can choose which words we want to hold on to. Words that make us feel brave and well and strong. "You're going to be just fine." Those words were medicine for my soul that day. In my opinion, it was as strong a medicine as any chemotherapy drug or radiation treatment in the world.

I walked out of there with the declaration that *"I will not die but live, and will proclaim what the Lord has done." Psalm 118:17* I'm forever grateful for this woman. May God give her an extra gem in her crown for that one.

Oddly enough, the months of chemotherapy and the weeks of radiation are a blur in my memory. However, what I want you to know is that the treatments were successful and I was eventually declared cancer free.

The lessons I learned during that time in my life are too numerous to mention here, but what I want to share with you is my conviction regarding the importance of consistent self-exams, the healing power of praying scripture over yourself, the peace that comes when trusting your own inner voice and intuition and the power of praying friends.

As you read further, you'll see how these lessons blessed me for what was to come. I pray they will bless you too as you journey through life, even when it may not seem so beautiful during times of uncertainty.

God is in you, God is with you, God is for you.

Dear Lord,

I believe with all my heart that you hate cancer more than I do. I thank you that amid the fear and uncertainty you were my constant source of strength. Through so many moments of anxiety, you turned me back to trusting you. Thank you for being with me. I ask your blessing on those who have had, currently have or will have to deal with this horrible disease. Guide them by the power of the Holy Spirit and heal them.

In Jesus' name, Amen.

FOR YOUR OWN READING: PSALM 118

8

I Can Feel You

"Death is a challenge. It tells us
not to waste time. It tells us to
tell each other right now that we
love each other." ~Leo Buscaglia

M Y MOM LOST HER ELDEST DAUGHTER AND
my siblings and I lost our sister Maria on May 4, 2016.
She died of lung cancer at the age of 63. It was without
a doubt one of the worst days of my life.

I always thought she would outlive all of us. I truly did.
She was so strong. So tough in mind and spirit and body. I
didn't get to vote. She's gone.

I'll never forget the conversation she had with her oncologist as she was dying. She was surrounded by her family at
our local hospital, and he said to her, "Maria, are you scared?"

Without pause she said, "No."

He said, "What do you feel?"

"Sad," she said.

My heart broke in two.

I knew why she wasn't scared, and I knew why she was sad. She believed that without a doubt she was going to be with Jesus. There was no doubt in her mind about that. We talked at great length about it and she was clear. However, she was extraordinarily sad that she wouldn't be able to be with her daughter and her grandchildren as they continued to grow.

"He will wipe every tear from their eyes. There will be no more death or mourning or crying or pain, for the old order of things has passed away." ~Revelation 21:4

I knew Maria as well as she knew herself. That's a real God wink, since as kids we couldn't have been more different. She was grown up before her years and I was a geeky kid beyond mine. We were only three years apart, but to look at us when she was 13 and I was 10, you would have thought she was my mother.

Maria was a very private person. She gave everything she had to those she let in and to anyone who was truly in need. She was generous, fiercely loyal, funny, adventurous, rebellious in her youth, extraordinarily smart and confident, physically strong and beautiful. She loved deeper than anyone I have ever known.

She never judged. She had remarkable intuition. She was an avid reader. She took chances.

When she got sick, she suffered greatly for three years. Still, she was courage on legs. Now she's with Jesus. I just know he adores her; I know he loves her hugs.

I was looking at a picture of her the other day and I could feel her. I could feel the way her strong hands would hold mine. I could feel the hugs she would give me, always the last to let go. I could feel her skin and how soft it was. I could feel her hand cup my face and tell me that I was beautiful.

She created a nickname for the two of us. It was Simon. It was based on the story in the Bible when Simon carried the cross for Jesus when he couldn't carry it any further. One day she started calling me Simon. For some reason, I reciprocated and started calling her Simon right back. This name that we used between the two of us didn't mean that we loved each other more than others. It was just us. It was one of those things that fit our relationship and stuck with us both until she died.

"Contented with little, yet wishing for more."
~Charles Lamb

Since she's been gone, I often reflect back on how much she helped me in my journey in life. I can still feel her in my memories. I still lean into what we shared, and it helps me carry on.

I miss her every day. I long for the deep conversations we used to have. I miss having her to listen to me vent, and I trusted her completely. Only she knew how much.

I wish I could have seen her as she entered into glory. I just know she finally received the praise, glory and honor she so richly deserved. I'm grateful Lyle got to see it.

My Simon, I hope you're standing at the gates with Jesus to greet me when I get to heaven. No one hugs like you.

Who is your Simon? If you can answer this question, I would encourage you to put this book down and call her (or him) right now and say, "Thank you."

Heavenly Father,
Thank you for my sister Maria, my Simon. You know how much she meant to me yet I know she is at home in heaven with you. I pray that each of your children can find a Simon who knows them and loves them like Maria loved me.
In Jesus' name, Amen.

FOR YOUR OWN READING: 1 PETER 1, REVELATION 21

9

Sometimes You Just Have to Be Brave

"Being brave doesn't mean we have no fear; it means we refuse to be overcome by it." ~Steven Furtick

FOUR YEARS LATER, AS I LAY THERE IN THE darkness of my bedroom, I did a self-breast exam, just as I had done nearly every week, if not more often, since my original breast cancer diagnosis and treatments.

I felt another lump. Different breast, different location. Same knowing. It was not there the week before. My heart sank, and I whispered, "Oh, my God, no."

The next morning, I immediately made an appointment with my regular M.D. The details that followed are so blurred that I can't articulate the order in which things transpired. All I remember is that I had to have a biopsy and it turned out to be Stage 1 breast cancer again.

I was sent to a surgeon, and he did a physical exam. He couldn't feel it, but he knew it was there from the biopsy. He sent me to an oncologist, who gave me a physical exam. She couldn't feel the lump, but she knew it was there from the biopsy. I could feel it because I know my own body. It was that small.

The surgeon and the oncologist both recommended I do the same protocol that I had been through four years earlier. Because I had been through it before, I knew the path that lay ahead of me if I chose to go that way again.

In every way imaginable this new surgeon and this new oncologist were completely different than those who had treated me previously. The diagnosis was the same and the suggested protocol was the same, but they were not.

From the moment I spoke with each of them, they allowed me to cry, to express my faith, to feel fear and ultimately surrender to whatever choices I wanted to make.

The surgeon said to me, "Thea, you are the boss here, not me. I'm here for you. I've told you what I think and I'm backing it up with everything I know. I will do everything I can for you, and I believe that you will be healthy because of it. You tell me what you choose to do, and we'll do it." Then he gave me his cell phone number and told me to use it if needed, any time, day or night. Yes, his personal cell phone number. He told me he would never operate on anyone who didn't have it.

The oncologist said to me, "You've been through a lot in the past six years. A lot of folks (I loved that this young southern woman called people folks) can't handle losing a spouse, but to lose him and then your sister to cancer, and then to be diagnosed with it yourself and now to be diagnosed with it again? That is a lot! You have an amazing attitude and faith. If you need to cry, you can cry. If you need to think things through, you can think things through. It doesn't mean you're not strong. You're entitled to your feelings. All of them. This is your body and your life. I'm here to care for you. I believe in the treatments I'm recommending to you, and I believe that you are going to get through them strong and come through them healthy. You choose and I'll respect your choice."

The only decision I could make at this point was a no-brainer, and that was to take the BRCA gene test. I don't think I ever prayed harder for a negative test result in my life. If I tested positive, my daughter and granddaughters and siblings would be at higher risk of cancer. The test came back negative. I felt like dancing. Actually, I think I did!

I then needed to get quiet and listen to God. So, I prayed. I prayed and prayed and prayed some more. I prayed for clarity. I prayed for wisdom to make the right decision. I prayed for God's grace to blanket me, and I prayed for courage.

The day before I was to give the doctors my decision, I was sitting on my couch with the TV on. It was during the day and I rarely, if ever, had the TV on during the day. I think I needed another voice, any voice that would be loud enough to drown out the one in my head that felt so scared and unsure. I was just sitting there numb, staring at something on TV.

Just at that point a commercial came on. It was a young girl, maybe 10 or 11 years old. She was bald. She was in a surgical gown, sitting on a hospital bed. It was a commercial for St. Jude Children's Hospital, one of my favorite charities. The only thing she said was, "Sometimes you just have to be brave."

I wept. Right then and there I decided to be brave.

I did the protocol, covering myself through each treatment in prayers of healing that I had memorized. I prayed the same prayers of healing over my body and my life that I had used back then. I still pray those same prayers today. With gratitude beyond anything I can describe to you, by God's grace I was once again declared cancer free.

I knew that God was with me when I felt something no one else could feel. I know that he is with me now. He whispers to me to be easier on myself. To be careful with the people with whom I surround myself. To pay attention to words and people who create dis-ease in me. To allow the blessed Holy Spirit to minister his peace to my soul.

Dis-ease. I cannot afford to be in that state, and neither can you.

Dear Heavenly Father,

Thank you for helping me choose to be brave when I was so scared. Thank you for guiding me and counseling me. Thank you for clarity when I get quiet enough to listen and thank you for protecting me from dis-ease. I need you, Lord, every single day.

In Jesus' name, Amen.

FOR YOUR OWN READING: PSALM 119

10
Dealing with the Hits

"Your hardest times often lead
to the greatest moments in
your life." ~Roy T. Bennett

A S I WROTE THIS, I LONGED FOR THE DAYS OF unquestionable confidence, when I had an innate and unwavering faith that life is good, people are good and that happily ever after was a certainty.

I discovered that my confidence started returning to me through measurable though oftentimes small successes. That's why it was crucial to take action on the very things that caused my heart to pound and my throat to feel like it was closing up.

The greatest reward of taking action in the face of fear was how much I leaned on God and his Word during those times. It forced me within, to a place of faith. "*For the word of God is alive and active. Sharper than any double-edged sword, it penetrates even to dividing soul and spirit, joints and marrow; it judges the thoughts and attitudes of the heart.*" Hebrews 4:12

It can cut two ways when used by a gifted swordsman. The Word of God has always enabled me to separate the lie of fear from the truth of whom God created me to be and how to live. *"For the Spirit God gave us does not make us timid, but gives us power, love and self-discipline." 2 Timothy 1:7*

As I mentioned earlier, three months after my guy died of lung cancer, my sister Maria was diagnosed with the same disease. About a year after that, I was diagnosed with breast cancer for the first time. My sister and I both lost our hair and sported wigs. We both hated cancer, but she had always loved wigs. In fact, she looked gorgeous in them, sophisticated even. Me? Not so much. I only wore them while working because I thought others might feel more comfortable around me. Others could see me, of course, just not my very bald head. Eventually, I switched to wearing beanies instead of a wig. Maria stayed with her beautiful wigs.

"We wouldn't worry so much about what others think of us, if we realized how seldom they do." ~Eleanor Roosevelt

The second time around, I refused to wear a wig at all. I wore ball caps or beanies or showed my bald head to the world. Funny thing is, no one seemed to care!

My beautiful sister died three years later. I was in an unspeakable and impenetrable fog.

Yet, by God's amazing grace and my fervent belief in self-exams, I caught the lumps early both times. Both my diagnoses were Stage 1 with nothing in my lymph glands. The second time around I was tested for the BRCA gene. Came back negative. Praise God! It was one thing to go through it myself, but it was terrible to think that my daughters and granddaughters could inherit this from me or that my other sister and her daughters might have to get checked. I don't think I ever prayed harder.

I chose to undergo chemotherapy and radiation both times. I had many people tell me they would never do that, no matter what. That was hard for me to hear. It was already a vulnerable time and the decisions were difficult to make. In the end, I did what was best for me and what I could live with.

I share this with you only to help you understand that during these times, not only did I take an emotional hit, but my professional confidence took a hit as well. A big hit. The world as I knew it had been turned upside down and inside out. I functioned in a state of what I called emotional Novocain for an exceedingly long time.

I've mentioned that I'm a verbal processor. It's how I work things out in my mind. I can hear myself talking out loud and literally get answers to my own questions. I think this is why people go to therapy. To talk things out. To hear things out loud and have someone listen who will not judge, but rather facilitate solutions. Bill, a dear friend of mine, shared a phrase with me years ago when I was verbally processing with him. "T," he said, "we have the answers, we just don't know what the questions are."

Lyle and Maria knew what the questions were for me. They were the ones I always went to when I needed to process out loud. This often allowed me to appear stronger than I really was to those who needed me to be strong, like my daughter and those that I led in business. I could talk to Lyle or Maria and get clarity, let things go, and come back stronger than I was before we had our conversations. I always appreciated that. Until they were both gone, I had no idea how much I depended on them, relied on them and got strength from them.

I don't know about you, but God has yet to physically sit and have a cup of coffee or a glass of wine with me and listen to me verbally process.

In the end, I tried grief therapy. I went to two different women. Both were lovely, skilled and kind. However, they weren't the answer for me.

God was my answer then and remains my answer now. He was about to teach me that he was with me wherever

I went and that his grace was sufficient, even for a verbal processor like me.

The Apostle Paul understood this as well as anybody when he wrote to his friends in Corinth: *"My grace is sufficient for you, for my power is made perfect in weakness. Therefore, I will boast all the more gladly about my weaknesses, so that Christ's power may rest on me." 2 Corinthians 12:9*

After this nudging by the Holy Spirit, I dug into God's Word more voraciously than before. I began to study Bibles that I wouldn't have read prior to Lyle's diagnosis, mostly due to the depth of the commentaries. I suddenly couldn't get enough. The only comfort I felt was from God's word. It was alive and life-giving. It helped drain my self-pity and urged me to keep going even when I felt like I was walking in quicksand.

I am in no way saying that therapy isn't a good thing. Not at all! I learned a lot and I'm grateful I went. It gave me a safe space to cry without putting more pressure on those with whom I'm close. Ultimately, it was not the answer for me.

I miss my husband. I miss my sister. I'll never stop missing them as long as I'm alive. However, God has met me at the center of every trial, every fear, every sadness. He has sustained me through all my loneliness and every moment of my grief. His Word whispers secrets to me. He gives me moments of joy and peace. He bolsters and sustains my faith. He goes before me. He stands beside me. He never forsakes me. I hold him close while I visualize him holding me. He's my best friend. One day I plan to have that cup of coffee or glass of wine with Jesus, as he sits and listens to me go on and on. I hear he saves the best for last.

Dear Lord,

Thank you that in the absence of Maria and Lyle, you have filled that space of loss with dear friends and family who really love me, care for me, are kind to me, patient with me and listen to me. They have been a comfort and a blessing. Thank you, living and eternal King, for you have mercifully restored my soul within me. Great is your faithfulness.

In Jesus' name, Amen.

FOR YOUR OWN READING: JOSHUA 1, 2 CORINTHIANS 12

Remembering the Light

11

God's Timing

"God's timing is magnificent!"
~Laila Akita

I BELIEVE IN GOD'S PERFECT TIMING, BUT ON THE day Lyle passed away, I wish I could have read what I'm going to share with you now. I have no way of knowing if it would have helped me get out of myself and continue to focus on my responsibilities sooner than I did, but I want to include it here in case it can bless someone who has experienced a devastating loss.

In sharing this piece, I am in no way inferring that grieving isn't necessary. Nor am I trying to tell anyone what the grieving process should be like for them. I'm not putting time limits on anybody's grief, and I'm not judging anyone's process. There's no course on grief except to be grieving, and I know for certain that it's different for everyone. I honor that with all that I am. I'm sharing it because what J.R. Miller encourages believers to be after a great loss, is exactly the opposite of who I was. As he mentions in his writing, my strength did change to weakness, and darkness had crept into my heart. When I was finally able to take up the tasks and duties to which God had called me, the light did come again, and I became stronger.

"Weeping inconsolably beside a grave can never give back love's banished treasure, nor can any blessing come out of such sadness. Sorrow makes deep scars; it writes its record ineffaceably on the heart which suffers. We really never get over our great griefs; we are never altogether the same after we have passed through them as we were before. Yet there is a humanizing and fertilizing influence in sorrow which has been rightly accepted and cheerfully borne. Indeed, they are poor who have never suffered, and have none of sorrow's marks upon them. The joy set before us should shine upon our grief as the sun shines through the clouds, glorifying them. God has so ordered, that in pressing

> on in duty we shall find the truest, richest comfort for ourselves. Sitting down to brood over our sorrows, the darkness deepens about us and creeps into our heart, and our strength changes to weakness. But, if we turn away from the gloom, and take up the tasks and duties to which God calls us, the light will come again, and we shall grow stronger." ~J. R. Miller

Ah, the beauty of words that can give life to the reader. Thank you, J.R. Miller. May your words continue to shine a light into the lives of those who are grieving, moving them into God's calling and toward his glory.

Gracious Lord,

I know your timing is always perfect; never early, never late. You know and have always known what is best for me. Thank you for loving me every day, even when I was living in fear and doubt.

In Jesus' name, Amen.

FOR YOUR OWN READING: ROMANS 5

12
I Have Got to Get a Life!

"To be a good mother while my heart was breaking was one of the hardest roles I've ever had to play." ~Unknown

FTER LYLE DIED, I BEGAN TO DEPEND ON MY daughter, her kind husband and their three amazing girls way too much. During this time, while she carried incredible responsibilities at work along with tending to her husband and three girls, I relied on my daughter to help carry my pain. It was unhealthy for both of us. I also turned into one of those grandmothers who unknowingly (I promise) tried to fill a void with the attention and affection of these amazing kids. Only recently have I come to realize this. No one is drawn to a needy person. Including me. I cringe when I think about how much I depended on them to be what I called my joy-source. Phew. It all happened so gradually. I had an inkling, but I truly wasn't aware that I had become so dependent upon them. I'm grateful their cheeks aren't permanently bruised from me smooching them any time I could.

Although I had the great joy of spending a lot of time with each of them as they were babies and toddlers, I forgot that while they were growing, I was grieving. The only way I could come to grips with this was by spending a lot of time with my own mother, Boppin' Bess. I'll tell you more about her later. At the time I wrote this, my dear mom had just turned 94 and was still living by herself. Most days she was in tremendous pain from arthritis and degenerative discs in her spine. Every day

"Motherhood is a choice you make every day, to put someone else's happiness and well-being above your own. To teach the hard lessons, to do the right thing even when you're not sure what the right thing is...and to forgive yourself, over and over again, for doing everything wrong."
~Donna Ball

I called her to see how she was doing. She would say, "I'm okay, honey. My back hurts, but I'm okay." Then she would immediately turn the attention back to me. "How are you, Thea?" she'd ask.

How am I? Yep, that's what emotionally healthy mothers say. "How are you?" My mom would then start laughing at something we were talking about, and when I'd hang up, I'd think, "Man, I just love talking to her."

I don't know for sure, but I would venture to guess that during the dark season in my life, my daughter had most likely hung up from me many times thinking, "Ugh, I love her, but, man, I wish she'd get a life!" She'd probably deny it, but it was not a good situation. I used to be the mom who had a full life, and who, I think, made my kid laugh. The mom who would intentionally strive to leave our conversations with her being lifted and feeling better and stronger and happier than before we spoke.

Thank God that through this awareness of my dependency, I began to see things shift back to who we once were together – back to a normal, healthy relationship where I was the mother, and she was the daughter.

I hope that my daughter and granddaughters know that I am truly more concerned about them than about myself.

I have learned through these experiences that it was my insecurity in the world that caused my dependence on them.

I have been determined ever since to find ways to fill my days, count my blessings when I do get to spend time with them and step into a life that will fulfill me while allowing God to continue to use me for his glory.

Finally, if you're lonely and needy and are trying and find a place into which you can plug your umbilical cord, I'd suggest not using your sons or daughters. It's not that they couldn't do this for you. In my opinion and from my experience, they shouldn't have to.

Dear Heavenly Father,

Thank you for my daughter and son-in-law and for my granddaughters. Thank you for helping me to see that I was putting too much pressure on them. Thank you for helping me find joy and purpose again. Guide me to the place where my dependence is on you and you alone.

In Jesus' name, Amen.

FOR YOUR OWN READING: PROVERBS 31

13

Head, Heart, Gut

"Intuition is seeing with the soul."
~Dean Koontz

A COUPLE OF YEARS AFTER LYLE PASSED AWAY, I had a phone consultation with a woman who, at the time, I thought was a grief coach. I thought this because her title literally was Grief Coach. I assumed she would deal with both my grieving process *and* how to pursue my work amid the grief. I was ready to move on. She was lovely and patient, but after 30 minutes she told me I was not ready to move on, and, clearly, I was not ready for her.

After asking me several questions, she told me I still had a lot of grief to work through before I was ready for her to coach me on setting and slaying new goals. She told me she only worked with people who were truly ready to get to work.

The interesting part was that I really thought I was ready and that I had come so far. I called her because I was hoping to get back into the swing of things.

I was counting on her to dazzle me with some blinding flash of brilliance that would snap me out of my funk. That would be a big fat no. There was no blinding flash and no snapping out of anything. To her credit, before we hung up, she gave me one brilliant nugget of advice. It was the only coaching she offered, but it helped me dramatically then and still helps me to this day.

Regarding the daily life decisions I had to make and the mental fog I was still in, she suggested that I ask myself these three questions any time I had a decision to make:

1. What does your head say?
2. What does your heart say?
3. What does your gut say?

She said to ask these questions of myself. My answers would reveal the areas in my beingness that were not in alignment.

My head, the logical part of me might be urging, "Yes. Go this way," and my heart might agree.

But then my gut would flag the deal and say, "Nope. Don't do it."

Or, my gut would say, "Yes!" while my heart or head would say, "No."

I learned to wait until all three aligned. Until all three said, "Go ahead," or all three said, "Nope." Sometimes the alignment was immediate and I would be clear as a bell about what I should do. At other times there was zero alignment, so I waited, prayed and sought the direction and leadership of the Holy Spirit.

To this day, whenever I don't follow this exercise, usually because of impatience or not wanting to cause conflict with someone who wants an immediate answer, I will sometimes decide to go ahead with an activity prematurely. Every time I've done this, I've regretted it.

Again, as a verbal processor it's challenging for me to make decisions without talking out my options. However, I'm realizing that the Holy Spirit is with me 24/7/365, and he will lead and guide me if I take the time to talk to him. He has yet to verbally answer me, but every time I ask, he does answer me. These answers come in many different forms: a chapter in a book, a simple unrelated conversation or merely a peace that settles over me. When I ask the three questions of myself and sit still long enough, all three answers align more quickly and peacefully.

What is your head saying? Think it out. Write it out.

What is your heart saying? Think it out. Write it out.

What is your gut saying? Think it out. Write it out.

Worth every cent I paid that woman, whose name, I promise you, I can't remember today.

I guess this process is the longcut to what Proverbs 3:5-6 suggests. *"Trust in the Lord with all your heart, and lean not* on your own understanding (head); in all your ways submit to him (gut), and he will make your paths straight."

I would encourage everybody to try this exercise. It will give you peace and counsel and help you make wise decisions.

Dear Gracious Holy Spirit,

Thank you for your patience when I forget to include you in my decision making, or in the joys or sorrows that life can bring or in my worship. Thank you for your counsel, which is always in alignment with the will of God. When I feel tired, I'm grateful that you never tire. Thank you for the gentle way that you call me into fellowship with Jesus. I'm thankful that you're always just a whisper away.

In Jesus' name, Amen.

FOR YOUR OWN READING: PROVERBS 3

14

Gratitude: Medicine for the Soul

"Gratitude and attitude are
not challenges; they are
choices." ~Unknown

W HEN I BEGIN TO FEEL ANXIOUS OR WHEN I
begin to complain, both of which stem from fear as
the root cause, I've learned that the only way out of
that state of being is to start thanking God for everything I
can think of. Out loud.

Philippians 4:6 says, *"Do not be anxious about anything,
but in every situation, by prayer and petition, with thanksgiving present your requests to God."*

Man! That is quite a request! Do not be anxious about
anything? In every situation, pray with thanksgiving? And
then present your requests to God?

That is some serious advice from good ol' Apostle Paul.

I believe that we all have angels who are assigned to us. The word of God says in Psalm 91:11 *"For he will command his angels concerning you, to guard you in all your ways; they will lift you up in their hands, so that you will not strike your foot against a stone."*

Yet, when I'm in complaint or when I feel anxious, my angels don't have anything to work with because I'm not in faith. It's my faith that puts the angels in motion. This state of being is caused when I'm being selfish or when I want control over a situation that is completely outside my control instead of focusing on God's grace and power.

This is how it goes: I'll pray, *"Dear God. You know my needs. You hear my prayers. I give all of this to you, Lord. I feel so anxious. I know you didn't create a spirit of fear, but of power and love and a sound mind, so please, God, help me. Send my angels to watch over me and minister to my spirit. Intercede for me, Jesus. Not because of who I am, but because of who you are. Help me, Father. Amen.*

I know God hears me. He's got it. He calls in the angels. They're ready to carry out my request in their supernatural ways. And then, I'll get lost in my own head. I'll take the corner of the prayer I prayed and hold onto it just in case God didn't hear me, and I'll try to handle everything myself.

Because God never wastes his grace, he gives a whistle to the angels to hold up. "She's not ready. She doesn't trust.

Come on back." And back they go. Ugh. I have no idea if that's heaven's reality, but I know this. When I pray without faith, I always become anxious and quick to complain. My prayers are ineffectual.

So, I begin to praise God. I thank him for everything. I proclaim and declare out of my mouth what I know he can do. I say out loud, "You did not give me a spirit of fear. You gave me a spirit of power and love and a sound mind." I surrender to the Holy Spirit, allowing him to shine in me. I stay in that state by staying in gratitude. I quote scriptures that affirm my faith and I pray again. I lean on my faith. I let go. The angles are sent in. I begin to feel peace in the midst of my storm.

Being thankful is my only way out of anxiety, self-pity or complaint. Try it. Just try it. If you're a verbal processor like me, it may take some practice because you might think that processing your thoughts and fears out loud will make you feel better. It will not. Cut your time in half and start with praise and thanksgiving.

Joyce Meyer said it best. "Complain and remain; praise and be raised!" Amen to that, Joyce!

Dear Lord of Faith,
For eight years I have woken up nearly every single day feeling fear as my first emotion. This

does not come from you. Thank you, Lord, for teaching me how to cast my fears on you. Thank you for the empathy this has given me when working with other women who are also filled with fear. I pray that one day this irrational fear will vanish. I know that no matter what I'm feeling, you are always with me. Cover me with your grace this day and fill me with your love.

In Jesus' name, Amen.

FOR YOUR OWN READING: PSALM 91

15

God Winks

"Always trust your gut. It
knows what your heart hasn't
figured out yet." ~Unknown

A S I WROTE THIS CHAPTER, IT HAD BEEN EIGHT
years since Lyle's death. Hard to believe. Sometimes
the days seemed to go so slowly, yet the years passed
by so quickly.

Every year around the time of Lyle's death, memories of my guy flood my mind. What I noticed this past
year was that the grief I once felt has evolved. It has now
turned to longing. Not the longing that I spoke about
in earlier chapters. Not at all. Before it was just a word.
Now, it's a feeling throughout my body that is tangible
and deep and all-encompassing. In my moments of longing (instead of grieving), my heart is filled with many
new emotions. They are intense, beautiful, emotional
memories. Delightful in a sense.

This change has taken much time and many tears, yet I now welcome these longings in my chest as an opportunity to breathe in my memories of him. As I remember to inhale deeply, I'll hold my breath for a few seconds while focusing on the pictures and the feelings that each memory evokes. Then I'll slowly exhale those feelings into my space and it's like having a treasured friend envelop me. At times, my tears even turn to smiles of thanksgiving.

These longings can be triggered by many things and often catch me by surprise. As I watch couples who are holding hands or laughing together or sharing a glance that they think no one else in the room sees (I see), I can recall with gratitude (and a sense of bliss) those same feelings without the pain of loss.

There are memories that I hold so close and are so clear that I can still smell the smells and feel the touches. A sweet caress, a tender kiss, a look of love. I still long for them. I still miss them. I know that I was blessed to have had them.

The week before Lyle died, he told my daughter, Jorgi, that he wanted me to love again, even to marry again. Jorgi told me this and she reminded me that I was sitting there when he said it. I don't remember it at all. I questioned her, thinking perhaps someone else was with them and not me. She told me the details of this memory were as clear to her then as when it happened, and it *was* me.

The subject came up again in a group conversation when someone asked me if I was dating. I proceeded to tell them that I had no desire to date. Jorgi was there during that conversation. It was after they left that she told me about the conversation between Lyle and her. I was stunned. I don't remember the conversation. Yet, it sounds like something he would say. It also sounds like something I wouldn't hear, since I was still in the fight-for-his-life mode.

I've heard it said that if you are in an unhappy or unhealthy marriage and your spouse dies, you likely will have no desire to marry again. If you are in a happy and healthy marriage, you likely will want to marry again. I'm not a psychologist, and I can't remember who told me this, but as I'm sure you can tell, Lyle and I had an extraordinary love for one another and an equally happy and healthy marriage. Still, I have not wanted to seek love again.

Within this longing for my guy, I've sometimes wished that I was open to loving again. Sometimes. In general, however, the longing that I'm feeling now isn't to be in love again. It's a longing for what I had with Lyle. Close friends have said, "No one can ever take his place, but you can love again and be loved again, just in new and different ways." I know this to be true. I've seen it happen to countless other people. I believe that most of them truly sought love again, and I haven't done that. Yes, I've mentioned it to God. I've wondered about it in prayer, but I've never asked him to find a man for me. It just hasn't been on my heart to do that. I've thought about it, but I've never prayed about it. That's noteworthy.

The other day I was reading the book of *Ruth* during my quiet time. One of my devotional books led me to that part of the Bible. As I read, I began to really think about Ruth and Boaz. If you don't know that story, check it out in the book of *Ruth*. It's beautiful. It's a description of how God became their matchmaker (that's my interpretation in the context of their story), and when he set them up, it was bound to be perfect. Their story is one of heartbreak, commitment, devotion, humility and restoration. It's a story that shows how Ruth and Boaz were separately, yet devoutly, walking with God in his perfect will for their lives. Then, during Ruth's pain and loss, love not only found her, but when it did, it was stunning and beautiful and filled with God's grace and blessing. Turns out that even the lineage of Jesus can be traced back to their union. It was literally a match made in heaven. As I read this story, it stirred something in me that was different than the other times I'd read it. I asked God what this stirring meant.

Later that day I felt compelled to share this story with my mom. She was familiar with the book of *Ruth*, so we talked about it for a bit. I went back to my computer and she continued to watch something on TV. Five minutes later she called me over. She said, "Thea, something just popped up on my phone (which she keeps right next to her on the couch), and you're not going to believe it." I looked at her phone and saw that it was something from Instagram, but from someone she didn't know. The Instagram handle was @ *waitingforyourboaz*. She read it to me.

It said *"One day God will bless you with one person who gives you everything that you've ever prayed and cried for, and it will be beautiful."* Mom immediately said, "Thea, this is not intended for me." We both laughed, and then I felt chills as I re-read the Instagram post and reflected on the tears that I had shed and the prayers that I had prayed on behalf of my daughter, Jorgi, after she went through a painful divorce. A friend of mine named Karen had shared a prayer that she had been praying for her daughter who had gone through a similar experience.

I started praying this prayer every night on behalf of my daughter: "Lord, thank you for giving Jorgi a beautiful man who will love her and her children and you as much as I do."

Every day for two weeks. Same prayer. About two weeks later, something extraordinary happened. She began communicating with Jonathan Madson, the son of some dear friends of ours. It turned into the most remarkable love story, and eventually they married. In March of 2022 they will celebrate their 10th wedding anniversary. He loves her and her children and God as much as I do. Jonathan was the answer to a specific prayer, and I thank God for him. What a beautiful reflection of how God works and moves in our lives.

Perhaps God is nudging me to open up to the idea of loving again. I honestly don't know. What I do know is that I love when God winks at my spirit. It's thrilling, reassuring and comforting. Loving one person again? I just don't know. What I do know is that God has something beautiful in store for me and each time my heart opens to love in any capacity, it's one more step in my process of healing. Yep. On this journey of life, God will heal our broken places and give us peace. Only he knows what that looks like for each of us.

I feel very blessed that even within my longing for Lyle, my fulfillment comes from my relationship with Jesus. I am clear that only he can fill my loneliness, no matter whom I'm with. I have felt him gently inviting me to spend more time with him, to get to know him more intimately. This has been a gift within my pain. I'm grateful that I'm opening myself up to whatever he has destined for me, love story or not.

Until that day, I'm happy with Eddie, my little Cavalier King Charles Spaniel, Boppin' Bess, my wonderful mom, my daughter Jorgi and her beautiful family, my close circle of friends, my extended family, my new love of writing and, most especially, the knowledge that Lyle is, and always will be, here in my memories.

Dear Heavenly Father,

Thank you for blessing me with many wonderful personal relationships. Within my longing for Lyle, my fulfillment comes from my relationship with you. This has been a gift within my pain. Continue to bless all those in my family and close circle of friends. My memories of Lyle will always be dear to me within these relationships.

In Jesus' name, Amen.

FOR YOUR OWN READING: RUTH 1-4

Growing Toward the Light

16
Love One Another

"Above all love each other
deeply, because love covers a
multitude of sins." ~1 Peter 4:8

LOVE IS HEALING. LOVE IS WHOLENESS. LOVING each other elevates us to the highest level of ourselves. And love, according to God's Word, covers a multitude of sins.

Think about that through the lens of God's love for us. Since God is love, we have the perfect model from which to build our own love muscles.

I'm sure you're familiar with the following passages, but indulge me as I share the parts where the Apostle Paul writes the following: *"Love is patient, love is kind. It does not envy, it does not boast. It is not proud. It does not dishonor others, it is not self-seeking, it is not easily angered, it keeps no record of wrongs. Love does not delight in evil but rejoices with the truth. It always protects, always trusts, always hopes, always perseveres." 1 Corinthians 13:4-7*

Verse 8 goes on to say, *"Love never fails."* If that's not enough, Paul wraps up this chapter with verse 13: *"And now these three remain… faith, hope and love. But the greatest of these is love."*

No wonder, love covers a multitude of sins.

When I started to really ponder this, my mind immediately went to our Lord on the cross, where he covered our sins with his blood forever! *"Greater love has no one than this: to lay down one's life for one's friends." John 15:13*

Because you love, you can then tolerate, you can forgive, you can bite your tongue, you can look for the good, you can accept each other's differences and you can sacrifice having your own way. Not easy.

It's easy to love the lovable. But the unlovable? Uh, not so much.

Even as I wrote this, I was overcome with thoughts of how many times I have said the words 'I love you' without fully understanding the true meaning and commitment behind them.

There are so many things you say you love, right? Your house, your car, your clothes, your furnishings, your accessories…but really? Love? Perhaps 'appreciate' would be a better word for all intents and purposes.

I reflected on my own feelings and actions in light of these words.

Am I patient? With those I love, yes. Otherwise, not so much.

Am I kind? I pray that I am.

Do I envy? Gratefully, rarely.

Am I proud? I work hard on this one, but, yep, guilty.

Do I dishonor others? Lord, I hope not!

Am I self-seeking? Yes, at times, ashamedly so.

Am I easily angered? Easily? No, but more often than I'd like to admit, unfortunately, that would be a yes.

Do I keep a record of wrongs? Truthfully? There are a couple stuck in my craw somewhere.

Do I delight in evil? Never! Just sayin'.

Do I rejoice in the truth? Yes! Rejoice!

Do I protect, trust, hope and persevere? With those I love, yes. With those I proclaim to love? Not always.

Do I fail? Of course! All the time.

Well, that was depressing, except for one thing. God knew that neither I nor anybody else could ever fully love. Not like he loves. That's precisely why Jesus spread out his arms on the cross at Calvary and said, "It is finished." He was showing his love for all of us. He was covering our sins with his blood.

Yes, God loves you. He loves you with unending love. Read the Apostle Paul's definition again and wrap your mind around the infinite miracle that is God's love. His grace is so abundant that it staggers my imagination at times.

In the meantime, keep this list of love descriptions handy. Read them. Ponder them. Work on them. Join me in rejoicing in God's love!

Dear Father,

Thank you for your unconditional love for all of humankind. Thank you for your patience when I conditionally love or when I don't feel love for others. And thank You for leading me back to the healing that love brings. Cover me in your grace as I learn to love as you would have me love. I can't do it without you.

In Jesus' name, Amen.

FOR YOUR OWN READING: JOHN 15

17
Nine Fruits

"The fruits of the Spirit are not
what we make ourselves do for a
moment but what God makes us to be
for a lifetime." ~Wayne Jacobson

A S A FOLLOWER OF JESUS CHRIST, I'M THANKFUL for many things. Yet, the Spirit who lives inside me as a believer is something for which I'm especially grateful.

We all know that the fruits of the Spirit are love, joy, peace, patience, goodness, kindness, gentleness, faithfulness and self-control. As a forgiven sinner, I'm clear that just because I have these gifts of God's Spirit in me, it doesn't mean I always allow these fruits to rule the day or that I display the character of a life submitted to God. In fact, I consider it a good day when I can reflect on it and be content that only by God's grace, and a good dose of his Word, am I able to live out some of these fruits in my decisions, behaviors and choices.

The late Zig Ziglar used to say, "Life is tough, but the tougher you are on life, the easier it is on you." It's never been truer than it is today. Life is tough, and people are hurting. And hurting people have a tendency to hurt others.

However, it's also true that healing people heal others. Therefore, I try to think about the fruits of the Spirit every day. When focused on and set as a priority for living, they mend and heal broken hearts while revealing a clear picture of how to live during difficult times.

> "He will wipe every tear from their eyes. There will be no more death or mourning or crying or pain, for the old order of things has passed away."
> Revelation 21:4

When I was much younger, I vividly remember committing them to memory, so that I could lean into them as a guide for living. I asked God to develop them in me, wanting to live a life that was pleasing to him. I wasn't trying to get God to love me more, as he already loves perfectly. (1 John 4:19, John 3:16) Rather, I wanted to please him the way one might want to please an earthly father. Not to get more love, but to honor him as his child.

As time has gone on, however, and I've grown older, I've realized what a gift these fruits truly are. They enable me to not only be as tough on life as I possibly can, but more importantly, to walk in my faith according to God's will during tough times. I need God's help with this every day, and he is faithful. I may not allow the fruits of the Spirit to flourish every day, but that's where free will comes in. The way I figure it, if it wasn't God's will for us to live by these fruits, he wouldn't have given them to us.

When do we need them the most? We need to love when we feel hatred stirring in our souls. We need joy when we are lamenting, sad or brokenhearted. We need peace when we feel overwhelmed by fear or lacking in hope. We need patience when everything in us feels like we are going to lose it. We need goodness when we are being mistreated and evil seems to be winning the day. We need kindness when we feel harshness coming at us and don't want to reciprocate. We need faithfulness when we experience disloyalty and when our convictions are tested or criticized. We need gentleness when we are on edge and our hearts feel hardened. We need self-control when we would prefer to follow our own will instead of the will of God.

It's easy to love when others love us. It's easy to be joyful when all is well. It's easy to have peace when everyone agrees with us. It's easy to have patience when we're not being tested.

It's easy to have goodness when others treat us well. It's easy to be kind when surrounded by kind people. It's easy to be gentle when nothing rattles us. It's easy to be faithful when others are faithful. Finally, it's easy to practice self-control when we're not being tempted. Sadly, that's not life on this side of heaven. Consequently, our Creator generously puts these fruits in us so we can rise to his calling. It's nothing short of amazing.

Yes, the fruits of the Spirit are a gift. They allow the light of the Spirit to shine through us. They draw people to us who are like-minded and counsel us when affronted by counterfeits. They strengthen us to not only live but to be a light for others. Each fruit bears more fruit, and while on this side of heaven, each gives us a glimpse of what heaven is like. After all, the Spirit of Christ is not only in us as believers, but in heaven as well, with the Father and the Son.

Dear Heavenly Father,

Thank you for the fruits of your Spirit. Thank you for your Word that brings life and for the counsel that I so desperately need as I face each new day. Continue to develop the fruits of the Spirit in my life as I submit myself to you. I thank you for protecting me when I'm weak, and for convicting me when I stray. Pour your amazing grace on me as I seek your face and your will. Thank you for loving me and for living in me through your Holy Spirit.

In Jesus' name, Amen.

FOR YOUR OWN READING: 1 CORINTHIANS 13, GALATIANS 2

18
The Dangers of Envy

"Envy is thin because it bites but never eats." ~Spanish Proverb

ONE OF THE TRUE ENEMIES OF PEACE IS TO BE around someone who has a spirit of envy. If gone unchecked, the fallout from this emotion can be confusion and discomfort. Envy has the potential to destroy relationships because it's difficult to trust an envious person. Without trust, there is no authenticity, for fear of judgement. Without authenticity, there is no real relationship. It's fake and superficial at best, with words needing be measured and weighed.

For me, envy is easily and instantly recognizable. A mental red flag pops up and my immediate reaction is to disengage as fast as possible. This adds fuel to the fire of an insecure person, which makes it even more sensitive to deal with.

There is an unpalatable feeling that shifts the soul of a person being envied and a sorrowful 'I'm not enough' energy that radiates from the space of the one who is feeling envious.

Envy usually shows itself in a passive aggressive way, since the real culprit is an unwillingness to admit admiration, in fear that one may not measure up to whom they admire. The victims of such emotions are ultimately insecure, living in a state of comparison. I can picture Satan smiling as relationships are poisoned in this colorless and odorless way, and it fires up my holy anger. Comparison is the thief of joy and the beginning of envy. It's an absolute waste of time and a tool of the devil.

> "Let each one examine his own work. Then he can take pride in himself and not compare himself with someone else."
> ~Galatians 6:4.

To deal with one who is envious of you, you can attempt to put out the fire of this toxic emotion by complimenting the person who is envious, building the person up or even expressing mild self-deprecation. Recognizing the insecurity, you can point out his or her gifts and blessings and encourage self-love. Of course, a dysfunctional and self-damaging way to deal with someone who is envious, is for you to put out your own light, so that the other person might shine more brightly. None of this works. Ever. It's exhausting with no rest in sight, because addressing envy without coming across as being arrogant or self-righteous is difficult at best. Even the greatest communicators in the world, and those who would seek God's guidance in their communication, will struggle to convey their feelings without coming across as judgmental.

So, if you are around someone who is envious of you, be mindful that it's a passive aggressive way of them trying to control you. Take caution and do not put your light out, hoping that they can shine. All that does is diminish the light of God within you. Instead, pray for guidance, clarity and most especially, pray for them. Give the situation to God, proceed to follow your intuition and protect your own heart.

As Charley Reese said, "It is never wise to seek or wish for another's misfortune. If malice or envy were tangible and had a shape, it would be the shape of a boomerang."

Instead, surround yourself with balcony people, those who are happy for your successes, gifts, talents and blessings. Those who call you to be the best version of yourself.

Yes, my friend, comparison is the thief of joy, and envy is a hole in the soul. This kind of insecurity cannot be filled by anyone but God, and neither you nor I are God.

Dear Lord,

Help us to remember the words of Dr. Henry Cloud: "Giving in to controlling people thinking that you're being kind doesn't work. All it does is enable a pattern to continue." Show us the balance through your agape love.

In Jesus' name, Amen.

FOR YOUR OWN READING: GALATIANS 6

19
Listening

"Enough about me. Tell me about you.
What do you think about me?"
~From the movie Beaches

FRIEND ONCE TOLD ME THAT I CUT HER OFF while she was talking. Not only that, she said I did it all the time. I could sense her frustration, which led me to believe that she had been wanting to tell me this for some time and couldn't take one more interruption.

You know that feeling, when someone says something to you that makes you feel like you just got kicked in the gut? Yep. That one. I felt like I had been kicked in the gut.

My defense mechanism kicked into high gear which caused my internal offense mechanism to swing into action. I wanted to lash out and keep score and remind her of all the times *she* had cut *me* off mid-sentence. I literally could feel my face getting hot. Yet for some reason, I didn't react. Praise God for that!

After I got back to a reasonable emotional level, I said, "I truly didn't realize I did that. I'm so sorry."

She said, "That's ok. It's just that you do it a lot, and I thought you'd want to know."

I'm clear that in light of all that is happening in the world, this is an insignificant thing. Looking back now, I can see things better from her viewpoint. However, I mention it here because if you're not careful, the seemingly insignificant things in life, the ones that you act like you're shrugging off, when in reality you're just stuffing them inside, can be deal breakers, heart breakers, divisive and destructive. When added up and multiplied they can affect a lot more than your feelings. They can affect your attitude, your walk with God and your own inner peace.

Did it hurt my feelings to hear my friend tell me this? Yep. Did I feel like continuing our conversation? Nope. Was I painfully uncomfortable saying anything else in the fear that I might cut her off again? Yes, indeed.

At this point, I had a choice. I could jump in and tell her that she did the same thing to me, which at the time would have been nothing more than a tit-for-tat, score-keeping confrontation. Or, I could take a deep breath, pause and apologize. I chose the latter.

If you're thinking that I'm tooting my horn about what a wonderful, forgiving human being I am, think again. It took everything in me to pause. I was taken back. I wanted to put her in her place. Most importantly, I wanted to be right. I've learned a few things over the years. One of the simplest lessons I've learned is that there are many times when I've had to make the choice between being right or having peace in my soul. I can tell you for sure that at this point in my life, I'd much rather have peace in my soul than be right.

"People don't care how much you know, until they know how much you care."
~Theodore Roosevelt

Are there times when somebody has crossed my personal boundaries of right and wrong? Of course! In those cases, I'm not afraid to say something. Not to do so would be disingenuous or even cowardly. In this situation, however, I didn't need to be right. I just wanted her to feel wrong.

We continued our conversation for a bit and then parted ways. I thought to myself, "Okay, now how do I deal with all these emotions that were just evoked?"

I took it to my Counselor, the Holy Spirit, and got some sound perspective on it. His nudge led me to realize that from this hurt, he was making me aware of a potential blind spot in my personality. One that could perhaps hold me back from fulfilling my ultimate dream, which is to help women understand how much God loves them, flaws and all.

I got the message loud and clear. The fact that this person had cut me off mid-sentence many times had absolutely nothing to do with the lesson I needed to learn. I don't know about you, but that can be a bitter pill to swallow. To tell someone that they do what they're accusing you of doing just to feel right and make them feel wrong is tempting. It's a ridiculous foible that I was grateful to understand.

It reminds me of the story in John 21:18-22, when Jesus told Peter what was going to happen to him. Peter, in an attempt to change the subject, asked Jesus what was going to happen to John. Very bluntly, Jesus said to Peter, "*If I want him to remain alive until I return, what is that to you? You must follow me.*"

After time with God about this, I was able to go from defensive to grateful, even relieved. I realize that sometimes I still cut people off during conversations, but at least I'm aware of it now.

"The biggest communication problem is we do not listen to understand. We listen to reply."
~Anonymous

Because of this heightened sense of self-awareness, when I find myself cutting someone off in the middle of a conversation, I usually will catch myself and do all I can to apologize in the moment. "I'm so sorry!" I'll say. "I just cut you off! Please, go on."

Nine times out of ten, the person will say, "That's okay. I was finished with that thought anyway."

I've discovered that I tend to do this when I'm fully and emotionally engaged in a conversation and excited about what's being discussed. I've noticed that when someone cuts me off mid-sentence it's usually for the same reason – enthusiasm in sharing!

Hearing the truth about a character flaw can be painful if you allow it to define you. It took me some time to absorb this criticism and filter it through the lens of who I am in Christ. Yet, I can still change "from glory to glory" as I spend more time with him. His mercy is new every morning! I love that.

The following quote could not be truer: *"Getting wrapped up in ourselves makes for a very small package."*

Precious Lord,

Day by day, I thank you for teaching me to make it less about me and more about them. Ultimately, it's all about you and what you do in us and through us. Thank you for the hard-to-hear lessons that awaken me to being a better friend and witness through my listening. Thank you for loving me as I continue to learn.

In Jesus' name, Amen.

FOR YOUR OWN READING: JOHN 21

20
Marriage

"And the two shall become one flesh."
~Genesis 2:24

MY FIRST HUSBAND AND I ENDED UP divorced after nine years of marriage. He was a great guy. Kind of shy, really funny, handsome and talented. Yet, I knew before I married him, and I knew walking down the aisle, that something was wrong. To be honest, I knew many things were wrong. Still, I rationalized (rational lies) it all, convincing myself that I could make it work and everything would change. I ignored the red flags, and I suspect he did too.

The beauty of God, however, is that he can take a mess and turn it into his message. He took two mismatched, naïve human beings and through us created our beautiful daughter and ultimately my three granddaughters. Beauty from ashes.

I'm not telling you this story because I'm an expert at love, obviously. However, I do know the difference between having doubts and having no doubts that whom you are about to marry is the one or not.

This might sound dramatic, but I genuinely believe that if you plan to marry, 99.9% of your happiness will depend upon whom you marry. Yes, 99.9%. Being married for life is a long time. I'm not talking just about commitment here. I'm talking about happiness. I know many people who would never get divorced based solely on commitment, but who are not happy.

I've observed that when a couple gets divorced, it usually has something to do with a red flag they ignored while dating, which escalated after the wedding. This was certainly true for me. The idea that things will get better after marriage is rarely true. Actually, the red flags tend to get worse, or at least our perceptions of them do.

I understand that many issues can arise that lead to divorce. Most of the time, however, I believe people fail to ask the right questions before they get married. I know with absolute certainty that if I had asked the questions of myself that I'm going to share below, I wouldn't have married my first husband. There's zero doubt in my mind about that.

If you have even one doubt, one tiny seed of doubt about whom you're going to marry, I would suggest that you pray and wait.

Be specific about what you're asking God to reveal to you. You will know in your gut if it's the right thing to do. After all, the gut is the second brain. I promise.

Ask yourself the following questions: (It doesn't matter if you're a man or a woman.)

- ✓ Do I like myself more when I'm with him/her?
- ✓ Do I respect him/her?
- ✓ Do I trust him/her?
- ✓ Does he/she have integrity?
- ✓ Would I be proud that when I'm not around, he/she is representing me?
- ✓ Can I imagine my life without him/her?
- ✓ Can we, and do we, pray together about everything?

Look, there are no guarantees that a marriage will last, but when you can answer all of the above with certainty and when you both have the mentality that "If you ever leave me, I'm going with you," chances are great that you will weather every storm and be married for life.

'Until death do us part' and 'in sickness and in health' are no joke. To fulfill these promises it takes certainty and the grace of God.

When dating someone, be sure to ask the following question: "If you were to mess this up, how would you do it?"

They'll tell you every time. If they don't intend to ever mess it up, they'll tell you that too. Try it. I'm not kidding. It's unreal.

> Dear Lord,
>
> Thank you for the blessings of marriage. I pray for those who are married and for those contemplating marriage. Help them to seek your wisdom, guidance and protection. Your Word says that two is better than one. Bless each marriage today and always.
>
> In Jesus' name, Amen.

FOR YOUR OWN READING: GENESIS 2

21

Pressure

"Pressure brings us to the end of
ourselves so that God can work."
~Unknown

ONCE HEARD THAT PRESSURE IS AN ILLUSION.
I'm not talking about physical pressure, like when you
think you can bench press a certain weight and the bar-
bell and weights come crashing down on you. That's not an
illusion, and, by the way, get a spotter. Sheesh! I'm talking
about the pressure you feel when you're under mental or
emotional stress.

To be clear, I'm not talking about the pressures that
some souls in the world are under. People who are not
allowed freedoms; people who are imprisoned or even
beheaded for their beliefs. I'm talking about the pressures you face on a day-to-day basis like family issues,
financial distress, raising children, caring for aging parents, health issues and so on.

When I first heard this, I was under what I considered to be a lot of pressure at the time. I was dealing with a situation where I had to make a difficult decision with lifelong implications, and I found myself thinking about it more than praying about it.

I had yet to hear the line, "Have you prayed about it as much as you've talked about it?" So there I was, ruminating, playing Holy Ghost, Jr., and getting nowhere, except, of course, to the licorice tablets for heartburn.

Then I heard this concept: pressure is an illusion. The pressure I felt I was under was all in my head and in my thinking. It was all in the way I was perceiving things. It was in the story I had completely made up in my mind. I had concocted a story and then unconsciously began collecting data to support that story. As a result, the pressure got more and more intense. This is what happened to me when I forgot I had a heavenly Father.

Finally, it dawned on me. I needed to make up a new story! I could decide right then and there that no matter the outcome, God would carry me. No matter the outcome, the promise God gave me was exactly that, a promise. *"For I know the plans I have for you," declares the Lord, "plans to prosper you and not to harm you, plans to give you hope and a future." Jeremiah 29:11*

I started to think back on all the times that he had guided

me after I had gotten out of my own head long enough to hear him. I began to dwell on his promises, and I remembered that *"Surely your goodness and love will follow me all the days of my life." Psalm 23:6*

The word 'decide' is based on the root word 'cide,' which means to cut off or kill off all other options.

In that moment of clarity I projected a new story into the hours and days ahead of me. The pressure I had conjured up around making this decision completely disappeared. I mean completely.

I began to breathe deeply again, and I began to get excited about the possibilities that lay ahead, regardless of the choice that I had to make in that moment.

Here's the part I want you to understand. Once I changed my story, no matter what came at me, I could see it through the filter of my new story. Then, each time I got more news or more advice, (the data I was talking about), I would listen through that filter. The pressure was off and I just needed to continue to listen to God's leading, do the next best thing I could do and trust him.

It's easy to say, but I sincerely believe that you will be as happy or stressed or pressured as you make up your mind to be. It's the making-up-your-mind part that adds the colorless and odorless sting to this. Oftentimes, before you even consciously know that you feel pressured and that you can change things by changing the way you think about the situation, you're deep in the throes of emotional turmoil. Your vision is skewed and foggy; your mind is confused.

This concept hasn't negated the reality of some awful things that I experienced. It doesn't mean that I don't still fall victim to rumination, which causes me to feel anxious and fearful.

Here's what the great Victor Frankel wrote in his astonishing book *Man's Search for Meaning*: "*When we are no longer able to change a situation, we are challenged to change ourselves. Everything can be taken from man but one thing: the last of the human freedoms – to choose one's attitude in any given set of circumstances, to choose one's own way.*"

Victor Frankel was in three different concentration camps during World War II. He lost his parents and his wife and nearly starved to death. He suffered unimaginable tragedy.

I read that Mr. Frankel survived these concentration camps because of his determination to finish a manuscript that he had started, which he believed would help mankind. There was intense purpose behind the pressures he lived under.

Jesus died on the cross at Calvary, paying a price that he didn't owe because God knew we owed a price we couldn't pay. While hanging there, after being beaten, mocked, spit on, taunted and humiliated, he said "*Father forgive them, for they don't know what they are doing.*"

Jesus, being God, was able to filter this human experience through the lens of paying for our salvation. It was his ultimate purpose in coming to earth – the purpose behind the pressure.

Pressure? An Illusion? Maybe. Purpose? Changes the story. Just a thought.

Father God,

The enemy of our souls is busy in our fallen world and we have much to pray for. The devil's greatest victory would be for me to fall victim to the pressures of life, to lose my joy, my faith, my hope and my belief that you have known my end from the beginning. Help me to remember during the times of pressure that there is nothing that can separate me from your love. Help me stand my spiritual ground during times of darkness. Help me remember that you love me and cover me with your protection every day.

In Jesus' name, Amen.

FOR YOUR OWN READING: PSALM 23

22
Working with Passion

"When you love what you do,
you'll never work another day
in your life." ~Anonymous

ON NOVEMBER 29, 1979, I BECAME AN Independent Beauty Consultant with Mary Kay Cosmetics. I was 24 years old.

I was blessed to be able to work my way up the Mary Kay ladder of success from Independent Beauty Consultant to Independent Sales Director. For the last 14 years of my career, I served as an Independent National Sales Director. To say that it's been a blessing to work with a company as unique and beautiful as Mary Kay is difficult to articulate. I will be forever grateful that Carol, my sister-in-law, recruited me into what I affectionately called our 'pink bubble.' Her mentoring, training, belief, work ethic and example of strength inspired me to work hard and to believe in myself.

Mary Kay Ash founded her company in 1963 on the belief that you should put your faith first, your family second and your career third. Mary Kay Ash was a devout Christian. She believed that when you put your faith first, everything else would come together. I agree with her wholeheartedly.

Mary Kay's system of priorities reminds me of a story about a little girl who wanted her mother's attention while her mother was on an important phone call. In order to keep her little one occupied, she tore a picture of the world out of a magazine, cut it into big pieces like a puzzle and said to her daughter, "Honey, tape the pieces together to make a picture of the world. By the time you're done, mommy will be off the phone."

She gave her the pieces and the tape and went back to what she thought would be a long phone conversation. Five minutes later the little girl stood next to her mother with the cut-up pieces of the world neatly taped together. Her mom was shocked. She said, "Honey, that's wonderful! But how did you put this together so fast?"

The little girl said, "Mommy, on the other side, there was a picture of a woman. When I put her together, the world came together."

Mary Kay believed that you should put your family second. This is something that I believe most people want to do. However, they may not work for companies that support this philosophy, Therefore, in order to provide for their families, they need to leave their families more than they like.

Finally, Mary Kay said to put career third. (Not thirty-third, but third.) Faith, family, career. I believe in this business philosophy with all my heart. It has enabled me to be bold in my faith throughout my career. It has allowed me to be there for my family when they needed me. It has allowed me to enjoy a fulfilling and rewarding career.

Here are the most valuable lessons I learned while in Mary Kay:

➢ Take care of your business when you can, so if you can't, your business will take care of you.
➢ A comfort zone is only a grave with the ends kicked out.
➢ People may disappoint you, but numbers never will.
➢ When others around you quit…don't.
➢ You become like the five people with whom you associate the most.
➢ Count the cost of your goals up front.
➢ Play now, pay later. Pay now, play later.
➢ Be willing to give up some things of comfort temporarily in order to reap the benefits long term.
➢ Success is about getting up just one more time than you fell.

➢ When things seem to be falling apart, the miracle is right around the corner.

➢ It's better to fail than not to try.

➢ It's okay to fall short but stopping short is hard to swallow.

➢ When things seem out of control, good things are happening.

➢ There are three kinds of people: those who make things happen, those who watch things happen and those who wonder what happened.

➢ Love is stronger than fear.

➢ When I throw myself into building people, the money will follow.

➢ Dwelling in possibilities is a decision.

➢ It's a choice to become bitter or better.

➢ Never complain about that which you allow.

➢ What you allow, you teach.

➢ The higher you climb, the more your slip shows.

➢ The higher you climb, the cleaner the air.

➢ If you don't want to be criticized, don't do anything.

➢ People resist an idea to the degree that it has power in their lives.

➢ Don't go broke getting rich.

➢ When you think you are losing friends because of your decision to grow, God has true friends waiting for you on the other side of that decision.

➢ Have an attitude of gratitude.

➢ Building a business isn't a popularity contest.

➢ It's nice to be important, but it's more important to be nice.

➢ Never take advice from anyone with whom you wouldn't trade places.

➢ It's fun to vacation in luxury, especially when it's free. Most people never do.

➢ Pain goes away when you win. It doesn't kill you if you don't.

➢ Life isn't a dress rehearsal and none of us are getting out of it alive.

➢ Play full out.

➢ As a leader, love is optional, but respect is mandatory.

➢ You can love people without leading them, but you can't lead people without loving them.

➢ Without integrity, winning isn't winning.

➢ Measure success by what you are capable of doing, not what others are doing.

➢ What people do speaks so loudly we can't hear a word they're saying.

➢ Hurting people hurt people; healed people heal people.

➢ Tough love is still love.

➤ There's nothing in this world that two can't do, when one of them is God and the other one is you.

➤ There is no happy ending to an unhappy journey.

Heavenly Father,

Thank you for the career I've been able to enjoy. Thank you for Mary Kay Ash, her life of influence, her belief in women, her grit, generosity and brilliance. Thank you for the mentors you placed in my life and for the many lessons I've learned while building a business. Thank you, Lord, for the opportunity to prioritize my life with you being first. Great is your faithfulness.

In Jesus' name, Amen.

FOR YOUR OWN READING: ECCLESIASTES 2

23
Desires of the Heart

"Desire, burning desire, is basic to achieving anything beyond the ordinary." ~Joseph B. Wirthlin

WHEN I WAS A YOUNG WOMAN, I WANTED TO be a famous actress. I mean world famous! The kind of famous where no last name would be required for people to know who I was. Elvis. Liza. Babs. Oprah. I could just picture it! Thea. Just Thea!

I didn't realize it at the time, but I didn't want to be a famous actress because I loved acting all that much. Although I think I had some natural talent in that arena, I didn't have a passion for acting in and of itself. Frankly, I wasn't crazy about the entire process. The memorization, the rehearsals and, dare I say it, most of the people whom I was around during that time. To me, it felt empty and shallow. It dawned on me one day that I just wanted to be famous for the sake of being famous. It would be nice for people to know who I was. It would be great to be wealthy and the center of attention. These desires, however, were ego-driven, self-focused and unfulfilling.

Looking back, I understand better what it was that I really wanted. The true desire of my heart was to make a positive difference in the lives of other people. I wanted to make people laugh, and I wanted to be used to encourage others.

It was during this time in my life when I heard actress Katherine Hepburn say, "Unless you feel like you can't live without acting, don't act!"

I thought to myself, "I could care less if I act or not." These thoughts followed: "What am I doing? This isn't a dress rehearsal, Thea! Find something you have a passion for. Something you would do for free. Then get so good at it that you'll get paid to do it."

Enter Mary Kay. When I started my career in Mary Kay and was able to speak in front of audiences, all the true desires of my heart began to be realized. I was in an arena where I could make people laugh while still making important points about motivation or business strategies or leadership principles. I could talk about how my faith has helped shape who I am and how much I rely on the Holy Spirit to lead and guide me. I promise you that I got on my knees before I would speak, asking the Holy Spirit to speak through me. I could study and prepare and then share and make a positive difference in the lives of those that heard me speak. It didn't matter if it was five people at a training class, 40 people at a sales meeting or 10,000 people at a company conference. It fulfilled me. It wasn't empty fame, and it wasn't ego-driven.

One day it finally hit me. This is my desire. This is where God has led me and can use me. I discovered that the word 'desire' comes from Latin and means 'of the Father.' Wow! Of the Father. Of God. Isn't that beautiful? It was for me desire expressed. If you have a deep desire for something, I believe that God put that seed of desire in you and has gifted you with everything you'll need to fulfill it. It may take time to develop your gifts, but they are there, waiting for you to step out, begin to grow them and then build on them.

As I think back on my work life, it's no wonder I wasn't fulfilled in the acting world. It wasn't God's plan for my life. I had certain gifts and talents that he put inside of me, but he didn't want me anywhere near Hollywood or Broadway. How do I know? Because I had no desire to go to either place. Only God knows what would have become of me had I pursued those dreams. I shudder to think. Yet, during my most courageous moments, I was able to use those same gifts and talents in the arena that I chose.

Yes, I went through a dark season in my career where I merely went through the motions. During that time, I stifled my gifts. I understand that now. I let fear win the day many times over, and I allowed dread to fill my mind. However, what I discovered was that the closer I stayed to the light, the more clearly I could see and feel confident that my gifts were still there. Whenever I did muster up the courage to surrender to the calling in my life, even in the midst of my pain and sorrow, I could feel the life coming back into my soul. This is what the dark side wants to prevent from happening. If God is going to use you, the devil will not be rolling out a red carpet for you. He'll do all he can to seduce you back to a dark place. That's why it's so powerful when you acknowledge your gifts and lean into them. More importantly, rely upon the gift-giver himself.

> "The great street of the city was of gold, as pure as transparent glass."
> ~Revelation 21:12

No, for me, desiring riches for the sake of being rich or influence in order to be the center of the universe were fruitless and unrewarding. The desire to be used by God for his purposes? That's what I'm talking about. The of-the-Father desires that led me to my ultimate purpose.

One of my very favorite stories is about an extraordinarily rich man who had only a short time to live and had a specific question for God.

Feeling that it was too much to ask God to visit him on earth, he prayed for an audience with Saint Peter, since that is who he believed would be meeting him at the pearly gates. His request was granted.

When the time came for them to meet, Saint Peter asked him what he needed to know. The rich man said, "I've worked hard my entire life and accumulated great wealth. From everything I've read and everything I've heard, I'm told, 'You can't take it with you!' I find this to be unfair. I earned everything I have fairly and squarely. I have tithed. I have donated. I have been generous to friends and strangers in need. I'm asking that I will be granted my request to take something that I've earned to heaven with me when I go."

Saint Peter said, "I will talk to God about this and get back to you."

A few minutes later, Saint Peter returned to the rich man and said, "God has told me that you may bring whatever you choose to heaven with you, but whatever it is, it must fit in one suitcase." With that he left.

A few days later the rich man died, and he met Saint Peter at the gates. Saint Peter said, "It's good to see you. I see you have brought your suitcase with you."

The rich man said, "Yes, I thought about it, and I decided the contents of this suitcase best represent all that I accumulated while on earth."

Saint Peter said, "That's fine. However, I must see the contents before you enter with it."

The rich man said, "Of course! Go ahead!"

With that, Saint Peter carefully opened the large suitcase to find that it was filled to the top with bars of gold.

Surprised, Saint Peter turned to the rich man and said, "You brought pavement?"

Quite the dilemma. All the material things of this world will be passed on. Christians understand that this world offers us nothing compared to what awaits us in heaven. Still, I've worked hard my entire life and had dreams of the trappings of this world. I believe that God wouldn't promise us a mansion in heaven and expect us to live in a chicken shack on earth.

Pray and ask God to give you the desires of your heart. Then, write down the answers to the following questions:

- ❖ What do I love to do?
- ❖ What would I do for free?
- ❖ What makes me feel alive?
- ❖ What can I do that will never compromise my values?
- ❖ How great am I willing to allow my life to be?
- ❖ How much is enough?
- ❖ What stretches me?
- ❖ What makes me laugh?

- ❖ What makes me cry?
- ❖ What gives me goosebumps?
- ❖ What puts a lump in my throat?
- ❖ What do I have a passion for?
- ❖ What can I do for the good of others that will outlast me?
- ❖ What gifts and talents do I have inside of me that are unique to me?

I've had a framed quote in my home for years. I don't remember where I got it, but I cut the quote out of something and framed it. It says, "Fall in love with what you're doing, and then get so good at it that people can't take their eyes off of you."

This isn't for attention; it's for excellence. That's how I want to live.

Whether you're nine years old or 90, may God whisper to you the desires of your heart which will lead to his will being done in your life. Ultimately, his kingdom will thrive and you will be led one day to an eternal home with him.

Dear Lord,

Thank you for allowing me to find the desires of my heart. I pray that those desires have helped build your kingdom and led others to know you and love you as I do. Your mercies continue to amaze me each day, and I'm grateful that I can call you Father. In Jesus' name, Amen.

FOR YOUR OWN READING: PROVERBS 22

24
Fear Not

"Fear defeats more people
than any other one thing in the
world." ~Ralph Waldo Emerson

D URING MY CAREER, I SPENT 90% OF MY TIME speaking in front of people. From the very first time that I spoke in front of a crowd of 600 people, I felt, and was told by many afterwards, that this was my gift. My gift was the ability to inspire, motivate and educate from a stage holding a microphone. For 33 years I absolutely loved doing it! I felt that God was using me, and I felt very fulfilled. It truly was my calling.

After Lyle died, I felt that my gift had died with him. I had no desire to be in front of a group and the times that I did speak, I literally could not feel my legs beneath me. It was a terrifying feeling. I felt completely out of control, but I continued to do it out of a sense of obligation and duty. Although the feedback was still very positive and women would affirm that I had moved them to tears or changed their lives, I couldn't wait to get off the stage.

At the time I wrote this, I had less than a year remaining before I would retire. Although the feelings of fear and anxiety that arose from speaking in front of a group had decreased, they were still there, and I was completely perplexed by this. I prayed before I spoke and relied more than ever on the Holy Spirit to speak through me. Sadly, however, I no longer enjoyed what I used to love to do.

I have worked with and been surrounded by many brilliant women over the years, all of whom are incredible speakers and trainers. To my knowledge, none of them ever felt what I felt. They were always jazzed up and ready to make a difference when they spoke, like I used to be. I can't tell you how I longed to feel that way again. For a long time, however, I just couldn't.

What I learned during this time, however, was that I loved to write. Writing is hard and time consuming, but I loved it! I'm my own worst critic, and I often questioned my abilities as a writer, but it was a craft that I took up with renewed passion and excitement.

When I shared this story recently with Gloria, a friend whom I respect immensely, she listened and said, "Thea, I believe that you are a gifted speaker. However, it doesn't matter what I think about that. Right now, if you want to write,

write! God will use that skill to lead you where he wants to use you next. Do what you want to do, and don't feel guilty about it!"

I didn't realize how much I would value that encouragement. I cherished her thumbs up and was happy to follow my bliss again.

I have unquestionable belief that God is leading me to a new chapter (no pun intended) in this next season of my life. More importantly, I believe with all my heart that through my fears, he has drawn me even closer to himself and his purpose for my life. The fear I felt was worth it. I know that now. It's still not always sunshine and roses, mind you. For me, it has been

"Of all the liars in the world, sometimes the worst are our own fears."
~Rudyard Kipling

frightening, so I keep reminding myself that God never said I wouldn't feel fear, he simply said, "Fear not."

I have taken that to mean that I can acknowledge my fear and allow myself to feel it without resisting it. The more I allow myself to do this, the faster I'm able to make fear disappear. Remember, what we resist will persist. Leaning into the feeling of fear eliminates resistance and it persists no longer. On the other hand, when I forget this principle, the more I resist it, the worse it gets.

The command to 'fear not' occurs 365 times in the Bible. That's one time for every day of the year. It's a serious command and worth heeding. I recently heard a minister remind me that if God commands me to do something, he will give me the grace to live it out. I bank on that every day.

I find it interesting that the Word of God does not say "tremble not, shake not, sweat not, have legs that feel numb not." Just fear not. Fear not!

> Heavenly Father,
>
> Continue to remind me that fear has no place in me. Remind me that fear can knock on my door but when my faith answers, it will flee from me. Thank you for your Word and for your soldiers of faith who stand boldly in the face of their fears, teaching me how to be strong. Thank you for the gift of faith. Without your power in me, I can do nothing. I feel your comfort amid my fears, and I'm grateful for your love.
>
> In Jesus' name, Amen.

FOR YOUR OWN READING: PSALM 3

25
Your Calling is Calling

"Fear knocked on the door, faith
answered and no one was there."
~English Proverb

W HEN I WAS KNOCKED TO MY KNEES PHYSI-
cally, emotionally, mentally and spiritually, it was
only through fervent prayer and God's grace that I
was able to stand up again.

Over the past eight years, I faced many fears. I also
discovered that fear wasn't something that could stop me.
There were plenty of times when I *felt* stopped, but the truth
remains that I was only derailed temporarily.

I felt it, acknowledged it and moved forward one step at
a time. God always met me in the middle of my fears and
calmed my spirit, rebuilt my trust. He was always there. No,
I didn't see him, but I know he was there based on the grace
that continually blessed my life. When I speak at events today
to follow through on commitments I've made, the grace of

the Holy Spirit always takes over and helps me get through my fears right in the thick of things.

I'm no expert, but from what I've experienced, God doesn't waste his grace. As J.R.Mueller said, *"God doesn't open paths for us before we come to them or provide help before help is needed. He does not remove obstacles out of our way before we reach them. Yet, when we are at our point of need, God's hand is outstretched."* I have found this to be true more times than I can count.

The evil one and those in the dark would be thrilled if you buried your gifts out of fear. Those in darkness are always out to cover your gifts and steal your joy. Your spiritual adversary is the father of lies. This I know for sure.

In order to honor God, I will recognize this and continue to believe that he has gifted me with many talents and abilities. In the end my joy is nonnegotiable, and I will continue to face my fears and use my talents as he wills.

Although I have allowed fear to stop me many times since Lyle passed away, I have asked God to forgive me for that, and I have forgiven myself as well.

I am once again allowing my deep desire to live full out the life that God has prepared for me. The desires of my heart are blooming again. My mind and spirit are joyful and willing again. "*I have brought you glory on earth by finishing the work you gave me to do." John 17:4* That was Jesus praying to his father. He completed his work down to the very last detail. Wow! Only Jesus.

As I connect the dots backwards in my life, I know that I've fallen down on the job many times. I also know that God has redeemed me from those failures and in most cases, used my failures for his glory.

As much as I've written about not giving in to fear, I'm not naïve enough to believe that I will ever be totally free from these feelings. As I wrote this book, I prayed continually that it would be a blessing to people. I prayed that my desire would be awakened and restored, despite the fear that used to cripple me.

As I mentioned earlier, the word 'desire' comes from the Latin language meaning 'of the Father.' So, if my desire is coming from him, feeling fear and doing it anyway is a no-brainer. I refuse to allow my past disobedience to keep me from using any gifts that God has given me to serve him and to be used by him and for him.

The Apostle Paul wrote: "*Not that I have already obtained all this, or have already arrived at my goal, but I press on to take hold of that for which Christ Jesus took hold of me. Brothers and sisters, I do not consider myself yet to have taken hold of it. But one thing I do: forgetting what is behind and straining toward what is ahead, I press on toward the goal to win the prize for which God has called me heavenward in Christ Jesus." Philippians 3:12-14* I too press on!

I remind myself daily that I am sinful flesh and blood, flawed beyond measure. Still, God loves me beyond my imagination anyway. I need his power and grace to fulfill any call he has on my life. That's why I lean on him so heavily. He does not tire. He does not sleep. *"The Lord will watch over your coming and going both now and forevermore." Psalm 121:8*

God doesn't force himself on anyone, but I can tell you this for sure. For every step I take towards him, he takes 1,000 steps to meet me. I believe he does this for all who seek him. There's not a doubt in my mind about that. *"You will seek me and find me when you seek me with all your heart." Jeremiah 29:13*

So, whatever you fear, move toward it. Chances are great that your calling is smack dab in the middle of that fear. You will be amazed to meet the Holy Spirit right there!

Dear Heavenly Father,

It seems like sometimes when I ask you to help me grow in my calling, it will start raining. Thank you for helping me understand that by this process you are grooming me into who you want me to be. Help me remember that every storm runs out of rain. Help me keep going even when I'm weary. Thank you for the reminders in your Word.

In Jesus' name, Amen.

FOR YOUR OWN READING: PHILIPPIANS 3

Transitioning into the Light

26

Friendships

"How you make others feel
about themselves says a lot
about you." ~Anonymous

F OR THE FIRST FEW YEARS AFTER LYLE DIED, I was invited to do things with a group of friends, to take trips or to just hang out as a group somewhere. More often than not, I respectfully declined. I didn't feel like I fit in. I didn't feel like laughing or dancing with someone else's sweet husband or rooming alone. The very thought of it made me feel anxious. As an added twist, I'm a recovering people pleaser, so I felt extremely guilty for saying no.

After a while, they stopped asking, and, strangely enough, I was glad. I began to realize

"Be somebody
who makes
everybody
feel like a
somebody."
~Anonymous

that I also had to grieve that part of the loss of my husband. I was no longer part of a couple. I was single – a widow. I had to feel it, grieve it, accept it and create a new normal.

I've come to learn that this is another small part of complicated grief.

However, the time came when I felt like I wanted to be invited to things again. Well, good for me. However, as I once heard, "People change and forget to tell each other." In this case, that person was me.

One day I said to Lisa, one of my closest friends, "You know, I get it. People just don't think to invite me places anymore. I've said no so many times that I'm not even in their consciousness anymore. I totally get that."

She said something that I'll never forget. "T," she said, "people think about you, they just don't spend their entire lives thinking about you."

Based on what happened to me, there was a lesson for me to learn in relationship to others who might be in similar situations. This is what I learned. If you want people to feel invited, or if you really want them to join you, invite them, and let them decide if they can go or not. It's not your position to try and figure out the ins

> "Be the person who makes others feel included."
> ~Anonymous

and outs of the struggles or pain your friends are going through. However, it can still be in your consciousness to stand guard over those you love. Unless someone tells you straight out to never invite them again, try not to assume, based on your interpretation of their lives, that they would not go. Even if they've said no a hundred times. If you want them there, ask them. The rest is up to them.

I have an inkling that this will save both parties a lot of mental stress, confusion, conflict and hurt feelings.

Side note and pet peeve: If you really want someone to be with you, please don't say, "You're more than welcome to join us." No matter how you cut it, it doesn't sound like an invitation.

Can you imagine Jesus saying to Peter, "You're more than welcome to join us." I think not.

I've experienced the phrase "you're welcome to join us" many times. In my humble opinion, it always sounded like I was being invited as an afterthought. I know it came from a place of politeness. Still, it felt disingenuous, hurtful and isolating instead of welcoming.

I would suggest that if you are inviting somebody to join you, try phrasing it this way: "We're doing something tomorrow. We'd love for you to join us." Which invitation would you prefer? Thought so.

Here's an example of a text I received from my daughter

one day while she was at work: "Hi, Mom! The girls' school is having an open house tomorrow from 1:00-3:00. I just realized last night that it's tomorrow. We would love it if you're free and want to come. I will be going right back to work afterwards, but I wanted to make sure you were invited. I would love to have you." I was all over that invite like a cheap suit!

> "Everyone is wearing a sign around their neck that says 'Make Me Feel Important.'"
> ~Mary Kay Ash

I'm confident that it took effort for her to have to stop in the middle of her crazy busy day and compose a text that made me feel included. Instead, she could have quickly texted me, "I forgot to tell you, but the kids have an open house tomorrow. It's from 1:00-3:00. You're more than welcome to come." Instead, she took the time to phrase it in a way that made me feel valued and wanted.

If you don't want someone to join you, for whatever reason, don't say anything. If a friend finds out about something and wants to go, it's up to them to ask if they might join you.

At that point, if you really want them to join you, you can say "I'd love for you to join us!" If you don't want them to join you, for whatever reason, you could say "I'm sorry, but it's not going to work out for you to join us this time due to (fill in the blank), but let's connect soon and do something together."

Let me add that if you're invited somewhere and for any reason can't or don't want to go, simply say, "Thank you! I can't go this time, but I hope you'll include me again in the future."

Am I nuts, or is this simply good manners? To me, the best beauty is beautiful manners.

Heavenly Father,

Thank you for the many wonderful friends you have placed in my life. Over time, they have become the gifts that I treasure the most. Help me to be a good friend to others.

In Jesus' name, Amen.

FOR YOUR OWN READING: ROMANS 16

27
Trust

"Do not trust your tongue,
when your heart is bitter. Hush
until you heal." ~Unknown

I WAS RAISED TO BELIEVE THAT YOU ONLY share your deepest thoughts and feelings, your 'real stuff' as I call it, with those whom you trust completely. To this day I've adopted this belief and practiced it in my own life. There are times when I gain clarity through verbally processing ideas. It's possible that people have thought I was sharing my innermost thoughts with them. However, I can count on one hand those with whom I've shared my real stuff. They know who they are. Thick or thin, middle of the night, weeping and fearful, lacking in hope...they listened to me, they held me, they listened some more, they lifted me up and, most importantly, they didn't judge me. They prayed with me and for me. I simply can't thank them enough, or love them more.

Trust is earned through experience. So is distrust. Not everyone has the personal compassion and empathy to listen without judging.

It's not easy to be trustworthy. It's a conscious decision. I understand that a crack can sometimes appear in the vault of confidentiality. Knowing this and having experienced this adds another layer in my bent toward privacy. My father once said to me, "If, in your adult life, you can count your true friends on one hand, you will have been a success." Yep. The older I get the more

"No one ever regretted the things they didn't say. Great minds discuss ideas; average minds discuss events; small minds discuss people."
~Eleanor Roosevelt

I realize what a treasure it is to have those few true friends who would "go to the wall for me," as Lyle used to say.

What seems more prevalent than confidentiality and trust these days is gossip. Gossiping is easy. It's also toxic and destructive. It's not only toxic to the listener; it's toxic for the one doing the gossiping. The listener can be sucked into listening, and that's bad enough. The one doing the gossiping has, in some way, already justified the comments in his or her own mind, and then willingly shared them. In my mind, that's the real tragedy.

A good question to ask yourself is this: "If the person I'm about to talk about was standing right here, would I still say this?"

I'm clear that personal privacy seems to be dying, especially in this age of social media. Of course everyone puts their best face forward on social media sites that others visit. Sadly, so much of what is posted creates a breeding ground for comparison. As I've said many times, "Comparison is the thief of joy." I've seen the damage it's done in the lives of people who constantly compare themselves to the unrealistic images they see in other people's lives. It's unsettling to say the least.

> "If someone is talking behind your back, there's a reason they're behind you."
> ~Sofia Brunie

If I could pass along three of the best pieces of advice concerning social media, it would be these:

✓ *Don't let the internet rush you. No one is posting their failures.*
✓ *Being famous on Instagram and Facebook is like winning at Monopoly.*
✓ *We live in an era of smart phones and stupid people.*

Years ago, the late, great Mary Kay Ash once said this about sharing your problems: "Half the people don't care; the other half think you had it coming to you." Cracked me up then and still does today.

In saying all this, let's be clear. I'm no saint. I've gossiped. I've broken the confidence of friends. I've judged others. I've been absent when others needed me. I regret each of those mistakes and try my best to honor the confidence of those who trust me.

It takes tremendous discipline to guard the words coming out of your mouth. The effort will always be worthwhile. If you're in a place where you aren't feeling great about yourself, or worse, when you think that by telling a story that isn't yours to tell, it will make you feel better about who you are, nothing could be further from the truth. *"For the mouth speaks what the heart is full of." Matthew 12:34*

"A gossip betrays a confidence, but a trustworthy person keeps a secret."
~Proverbs 11:13

You might be wondering why I'm sharing my real stuff here when I've always been a private person. It's only because I'm hoping that the real stuff I share might make somebody else's road easier. That it might offer a clearer map toward the love that God has for you. It's one of my constant, daily prayers.

As a final suggestion, know your safe places and never write anything down that you don't want everyone to know. I learned that the hard way. I've also learned this: If someone is talking to me about someone else, they are most likely talking about me to someone else. I know this to be true. This lesson has been a blessing and has taught me to guard my heart and my mouth when tempted to gossip or when I've been in the company of a gossip.

Dear Heavenly Father,

Thank you for allowing me and all your children to come to you each day in prayer. I am grateful that I can unburden my soul and feel your protective love each time I pray. Help me today to guard my tongue from gossip that I might be a blessing to others.

In Jesus' name, Amen.

FOR YOUR OWN READING: PROVERBS 16, EPHESIANS 4

28
Mom

"Will you still need me, will
you still feed me, when I'm
94?" ~Paul McCartney

A T THE TIME I WROTE THIS, MY BEAUTIFUL
mom and the matriarch of our family was 94 years
young. She gave birth to five children, one of whom
has passed on to glory. She has eight grandchildren and 14
great-grandchildren, one of whom has passed on to glory.
She has another great-grandchild on the way, one great-
great-grandchild and another on the way.

Until March 19, 2020, she lived on her own, ever since
the death of my dad. My parents were married for 50 years,
and my dad passed away at the age of 73. For over 20 years,
mom lived on her own. Until just a couple of years ago she
was mobile and very active.

Suddenly, she started to have some pain in her back and,
in a very short period of time, went from cooking, cleaning

and driving (even at night), to using a walker and living in constant back pain.

My siblings and I all lived at least 45 minutes from her and, although she had all the equipment to call for emergency care if she fell, we were getting concerned about her rapidly changing physical condition.

Let me first explain that when it comes to her mental capacity, she's fit as a fiddle. She occasionally forgets she's already told me something or what the password is for some app she's using, but she can beat the daylights out of me at the game of *Rummikub*, and she can hold her own with anybody playing *Words with Friends* or *Scrabble*.

"A kindhearted woman gains honor."
~Proverbs 11:16

For some perspective on mental capacity, the other day I was on my cell phone in my bathroom while putting on my makeup. The phone was lying on the vanity and I was chatting away on the speaker.

At the time, I was using a magnifying mirror to apply my eyeliner. Much to my chagrin, I realized that I needed to tweeze an inch-long hair growing out of my chin. Don't laugh, by the way. If you're over 50 you probably have hairs growing somewhere on your face too. If you think you don't – take a good long look in a magnifying mirror. Magnifying mirrors are from God.

Anyway, there I was, tweezing, lining, chatting. I needed to go into the other room to grab something that I wanted to share with the woman who was on the phone. So, off I went to the kitchen, phone in hand, still chatting away. When I asked her a question, I didn't hear her answer, so I said, "Are you there?" Still, I heard nothing.

As I walked back to the bathroom, I could faintly hear *her* saying, "Are you there?"

When I got to the bathroom, there was my cell phone, still lying on the vanity. My friend was yelling, "Thea? Are you there?"

Yep. I was walking around the house talking into my magnifying mirror. I put down the mirror, picked up my phone and told my friend what I had just done. We both laughed our guts out! Here's the point. Either I'm completely losing it, or my mom is mentally just fine.

Over the past few years mom has had a couple of temporary health challenges unrelated to her back that necessitated her staying with me for a month or so.

After this happened a couple times, I asked her to come and live with me permanently. Each time, however, after she began to feel better, she would tell me she couldn't wait to get back to her own place. She kept assuring me that it wasn't me she wanted to get away from; she just wanted her independence. I totally understood.

When things began to get worse for her physically, I asked her again to live with me. This went on for over a year, and for over a year she would say, "No honey, I'm okay. If I didn't think I could do it anymore, I'd let you know, but, for now, I'm okay. Please don't worry about me."

I tried not to worry, but I was concerned. I found myself calling her every day to check in, to make sure she was taking her medications and eating properly.

There's an interesting dynamic that can happen between a child and an aging parent. For the longest time she would call to check in on me or one of my siblings. She would just see if everything was okay and we would catch up. One day things changed. She stopped calling, and I started calling her instead.

She would always tell me that she was okay, but she admitted that she wasn't eating right and she was having a much harder time getting around. At the time, she was 94. Her spirit was willing, but her body had a mind of its own.

I can't begin to express the tug on my heart that I began to feel – the tug to care for her. One day, on our way back from a doctor's appointment, I asked her again to come and live with me. She said the same thing she always said.

This time, I said, "You know what, Ma? How 'bout I just come stay with you?"

Knowing her desire to be independent, I have to tell you

that I was surprised by her response. Without even hesitating she said, "I would love that!"

I quickly understood that she had finally gotten to the point where she realized she needed help. The only thing I insisted on was that when I bought a new home, she would come and live with me. She agreed. That's God for you. Always looking out for his children.

I knew this was a huge decision. Believe me when I tell you that I prayed a lot about it before mentioning it to her. In my spirit and in my gut the feeling to be with my mom had become so strong that it was like a constant nudging. Get up there! That's all I kept feeling. At the time I had no idea why I felt such a strong nudging, but I knew it was the right thing to do.

"She is clothed with strength and dignity; she can laugh at the days to come."
~Proverbs 31:25

Three years prior to all of this, I had sold the house that Lyle and I lived in and moved into an apartment. It was nice and safe and it was the perfect transitional place for me, but I knew I wouldn't live there forever.

Originally, I had planned to buy another house when my lease was up, but when mom started to have her challenges,

I found myself constantly making trips to take her to her doctor appointments.

Finally, I decided to ask the powers-that-be at my apartment complex if I could break my lease four months early to go care for her.

Normally, these apartments have a hard-and-fast rule that if you tried to break a lease early, you would have to pay for the remainder of the lease, even if you weren't living there. However, when I spoke to the woman in the leasing office, she said, "I have a list as long as my arm of people who want your apartment. I can't guarantee you that I can rent it, but I'm telling you, I can rent it. Give me the date you want to give your notice, and I'll list it immediately." I gave her my notice that day. She had it rented in 20 minutes.

I started packing immediately. My goal was to be out and living with my mom in two weeks. I missed that goal by four days. As it turned out, I moved in with her on March 19, 2020, the very day the state of California issued a stay-at-home order due to the coronavirus.

Prior to any of us knowing anything about a virus, God had laid it on my heart to go stay with my mom, and he wasn't being subtle about it. I would go back and forth with my list of what-ifs and my penchant for being a control freak, but God was persistent. I didn't actually hear his voice, but I felt it. I've learned that delayed obedience is still disobedience, so, thank God, I stopped thinking about it and moved into action.

I suspect you can feel and understand that I'm very close with my mom. I've loved her and respected her my entire life and have always considered her one of my best friends. The hesitation that I felt about going to stay with her was due to my wanting us to stay as close as we'd always been. I did not want to infringe on the independence that she still had. At the same time, I wanted to help care for her. It was a delicate dance. In the end, it was important to me that she didn't feel I was coming in to change her world or to take over.

Oswald Chambers wrote the following: "*It is one thing to choose to be disagreeable and another thing to go into the disagreeable by God's engineering. If God puts you there, he is amply sufficient.*" Chambers also wrote: "*There must be no debate. The moment you obey the Light, the Son of God presses through you in that particular; but if you debate, you grieve the Spirit of God.*"

These quotes seem to reflect perfectly the choice I made. By the way, there's nothing disagreeable about my mom. Nothing! She can be stubborn, but she's never disagreeable. In fact, if you look up 'agreeable' in the dictionary, there's a picture of her next to the definition. I got the message, so up I went to stay with my mom.

It's true that nobody knows what the future holds, but as

believers, we do know who holds the future. According to God's calendar, he wanted me to be with my mom.

The picture I had of my future did not include living with my 94-year-old mom when I was 64. It was not my plan to be stuck with a stay-at-home order hanging over our heads. It was not my plan to not be able to travel a bit, to get away once in a while, and still care for my mom. Nope. Yet, this I know. God's promise in Jeremiah 29:11 never felt more relevant. If I've learned anything, his promises are always better than my plans any day of the week and twice on Sunday. *"I know the plans I have for you says the Lord. Plans to prosper you and not to harm you. To give you a future and a hope." Jeremiah 29:11*

> "She speaks with wisdom, and faithful instruction is on her tongue."
> ~Proverbs 31:26

The sufficiency that Oswald Chambers wrote about became the very rhythm of our lives together during this season. I still shudder to think of her being alone during this pandemic. God made sure she wouldn't be alone.

Our living arrangement has had its challenges. As I've told you, I'm a verbal processor and mom is a stuffer. Because of this, we've had some emotional conversations. There have been moments when she would feel helpless as she watched me during a normal day working around the house, doing laundry, cooking, etc. It sharpened her focus on the fact that she was not able to do all these things any longer. It made her aware that she had lost some of her independence. These were tasks that she had done every day of her life as a devoted wife and mother, and now she had to have someone else do them for her. Although she told me many times how grateful she was that I was there, it took a toll on her to realize that it was just not possible for her do everything anymore.

Every day I feel God's grace which has allowed me to embrace this time with her. It's impossible to express just how profoundly grateful I am to have the freedom and the flexibility to be with her during this uncertain time.

The other day she thanked me for something I did for her. I said, "You know what, Ma? It's my turn to give back to you for all of the years you devoted to me. It's my honor to serve you. It's blessing me more than it is you."

Each of my siblings feels the same way about our mom. If any of them were single and living in close proximity to mom, I'm confident they would do the same thing.

When I came to stay with mom, I truly thought I was being called to help her, and in tangible ways, I believe I have. However, the help I've given her pales in comparison to the things I've learned from her.

At 94, she knows what really matters. She's learned not to judge. She's learned to breathe before she gets upset. She's learned to laugh...all the time! I'm not kidding. If I turn to her and say, "Shoehorn," she'll laugh for five minutes.

I play games with her and watch movies with her. I watch her play with Eddie, my furry companion. She laughs and laughs at his playfulness while ignoring his hair on her pant legs, and she does it all with such patience.

I just love being in her presence. I watch the way her hands move. I listen to the kindness in her voice when she teaches me something, whether it's how to cook or how to respond.

I've learned so much by watching the way she responds to life's challenges. It has literally changed me.

When I was growing up, like most kids, I didn't pay attention to how she handled her duties in the morning or her faithfulness in the evening. Today, I pay attention to it all.

One evening, after we had both gone to our rooms for the night, I remembered that I had forgotten to ask her something that needed to be answered before the next morning. I knocked quietly on her door. Being hard of hearing, she didn't hear the knock. I gently opened it, and there she was with her arms leaning on her bed, head down, praying. She used to do this standing up. I've roomed with her in hotels enough times over the years that I know this. Every night without fail, no matter where we were, this was her position before getting into bed. Because she has so much pain in her back now, she can no longer stand straight up to pray. So, she leans on her arms and elbows and prays. I closed the door and walked across the hall to my room wiping tears from my eyes. Character is who we are in the dark when no one is watching, but God sees all. I was glad to be in on that scene.

Yes, in isolation, we are not isolated. We have each other. For that, I'm grateful beyond measure.

I recently bought a new home and moved mom in with me. Initially, it was a difficult transition for her, but we've settled in now, and she's showing me once again why she's lived to be 95. She's back to laughing all the time.

In the trophy room of my heart, mom's trophy stands high. Don't let the old lady in, Ma. I love you!

Heavenly Father,
Thank you for granting my mom a long life on this earth. Her love for me and others in her life is a reflection of you. Her influence on our family and friends has been invaluable. Bless her and all parents this day.
In Jesus' name, Amen.

FOR YOUR OWN READING: DEUTERONOMY 4

29
What I Allow, I Teach

"When you have clear boundaries, you
permit yourself respect." ~Anonymous

A MENTOR OF MINE ONCE TOLD ME, "IF SOME-
one hurts you once, it was probably an accident. If they
do it again, it was probably on purpose. When people
show you who they are, believe them the first time."

Yes, you teach people how to treat you by what you tolerate. It's taken me a long time to understand this. As a matter
of fact, I'm still working really hard to create boundaries
while allowing love and kindness to lead the way. The idea of
setting boundaries is popular
in our society. "You crossed
my boundaries, so you're out."

"Forgive
people. Start
with the ones
who never
apologized!"
~Real Talk Kim

What's the real reason for
setting boundaries? And if you
set boundaries, can you go to
such extremes that boundaries

become walls so high and wide that there's no going back? Barriers that become divisive and unforgiving? That doesn't settle with my spirit at all.

Of course boundaries are important for your well-being, especially if you're being abused or harmed. However, showing love and kindness while setting boundaries reminds me of Jesus.

You can love people from a distance. You can forgive people from a distance. You can also be sure to not allow the boundaries you create to be so self-righteous that your own heart becomes hardened.

For me personally, I thank God that according to his Word, nothing can separate me from his love through Christ Jesus.

"When you're 20 you care what everybody thinks, when you're 40 you stop caring what everyone thinks, when you're 60 you realize no one was ever thinking about you in the first place."
~Winston Churchill

Follow your heart and the leading of the Holy Spirit. Remember this when creating your boundaries: "No." is a complete sentence.

Heavenly Father,

Thank you for surrounding me with people who build me up. My desire is to live in peace with all those that I love. Remind me today of your perfect love for me so that I can share that love with others.

In Jesus' name, Amen.

FOR YOUR OWN READING: ROMANS 8, ROMANS 12

30
Did I Just Say That?

"May these words of my mouth and this
meditation of my heart be pleasing
in your sight, Lord." ~Psalm 19:14

Y GOODNESS! HOW MANY TIMES A DAY DO I need to pray this? 70 x 7 apparently. Sometimes, it would seem such a luxury, a convenience actually, to not know the Bible and what God asks of his people. Then I could just rip someone's face off. (Did I just say that?) Aside from going to jail, there would be no spiritual consequences like being convicted of sin, damaging my relationship with God and having my prayers be ineffective.

It's unfortunate, but I have fantasized about this every once in a while even while knowing that I've been called to love. Called to forgive. Called to make peace whenever possible.

As a Christian, I understand that sin is always a lurking reality, a daily struggle. Yet, am I entitled to live my life offering only lip service while walking around in careless bliss just because I've been saved by grace through faith? Not so much.

If I know I'm a forgiven sinner but view that as a license to sin more, it's an abuse of my free gift of salvation.

Paul clearly recognized this when he wrote in Romans 6:1-4: "*What shall we say, then? Shall we go on sinning so that grace may increase? By no means! We are those who have died to sin; how can we live in it any longer? Or don't you know that all of us who were baptized into Christ Jesus were baptized into his death? We were therefore buried with him through baptism into death in order that, just as Christ was raised from the dead through the glory of the Father, we too may live a new life.*"

It's heart wrenching to see division in our country today. Whether it's disagreement on political ideas, social constructs or family ideals, without love and compassion, friendships can be destroyed and families disrupted. The dark side is loving it.

One of Lyle's favorite sayings was "If you don't stand for something, you'll fall for anything." I agree with that. It takes courage and forbearance to take a stand while continuing to love each other.

I pray for the day when people from all walks of life can take personal stands on issues without being criticized, censored or even hurt. Naive? Perhaps. Hopeful? Absolutely. May God's grace be on you as you seek that balance.

Dear Heavenly Father,

Thank you for the forgiveness you offer me each day. Each time I go astray, I know I can lay my sins at the foot of the cross and take the forgiveness that Jesus earned for me. Help me to be forgiving to others today.

In Jesus' name, Amen.

FOR YOUR OWN READING: PSALM 19

31
Abracadabra!

"Words can inspire and words
can destroy. Choose yours
well." ~Robin Sharma

I USED TO THINK THE WORD ABRACADABRA WAS just a made up word used for magic tricks. Then I discovered that it's actually an Aramaic word that means, "What you speak, you create." Powerful!

As beautiful as the experience was with the doctor who told me I was going to be just fine, I recently had an experience that once again proved how powerful words can be. Words that in this case were not positive.

Recently, the doctor that I had for years decided to retire. I was given recommendations for some other doctors in the area. I went to the first one and it wasn't a fit. Just different personality styles. No big deal. I was there a total of 15 minutes, and she didn't check anything on my body. Nothing. Gave me her opinion of what she thought I should do, much of which I didn't agree with, and I was on my way.

I made an appointment with another doctor. I liked him. He was young and very personable. He was kind and easy to talk to. We spent time discussing some things and he answered the questions I had. He asked if he could run some blood work to make sure that my electrolytes were okay. I agreed and had it done.

He called me back the next day to tell me that my white blood cells were a bit low, and he just wanted to be sure I didn't have blood cancer. What in the world? This was on a Friday, mind you. I told him he was freaking me out, my first natural tendency after having cancer twice. He told me he wasn't worried about it. What?

I said, "I'm going to call my oncologist right now. I'm not going through the weekend with the words 'blood cancer' running through my mind!"

For the second time, he said he wasn't worried about it, but he wanted to call and tell instead of contacting me through email. Oh my goodness! I felt like I was in the *Twilight Zone*! I mean, where was Alan Funt? Was I on *Candid Camera*?

As it happened, I was writing the chapter about my first cancer diagnosis the day he called. The chapter where I talked about how I needed to lean into God's promises and that even when I didn't know what or how to pray, the Holy Spirit prayed on my behalf. This reflection reminded me of all that God had seen me through. It reminded me that if the devil can't take us out, he'll try to wear us out. I knew I needed to fight his words with God's Word.

I called my prayer warrior friend to ask her to pray for me. I began to claim God's promises. I said them out loud and personalized them! *"The Lord himself goes before me! He will never leave me nor forsake me! Be not discouraged. Be not afraid!" Deuteronomy 31:8 "My God, I cried out to you for help, and you restored my health!" Psalm 30:20*

"Do all the good you can, by all the means you can, in all the ways you can, in all the places you can, at all the times you can, to all the people you can, as long as ever you can."
~John Wesley

I prayed for God's grace, mercy and healing touch and then called my oncologist. I was told that she was in clinic with patients, but she would get back to me that day. A couple hours later, her assistant called me back and said, "Doctor wanted me to be sure to call you right away to let you know that, based on your blood work, there is absolutely no evidence of any cancer in your body. You have nothing to worry about!" I could breathe again.

My oncologist called me after her clinic. It happened to be Valentine's Day, so she said, "Have a beautiful Valentine's Day and a great weekend. You're fine and we want you to stay fine!" She ended the call by saying, "I don't know why doctors do this kind of stuff. He's not a hematologist!"

I wept at *her* words, because I had been so frightened by *his* words.

To his credit, the doctor who had verbalized the words 'blood cancer' called me back that same day. He said he took the blood work and did further testing on it to confirm if I had it or not. (What a concept.) He said, "It all came back completely normal. I just wanted you to know so you don't go through the weekend worried."

I thanked him and told him that I had already called my oncologist and had received that news from her, but that I appreciated his calling and giving me even more confirmation through this test. But, oh my goodness! His words had scared the living daylights out of me!

I believe that even he knew that he handled things inappropriately and that he had scared me without proper evidence. I hope he learned something from it. I know I did. Words are containers for power. For good or for evil. For illness and for health. For life and for death.

Doctors, be sure before you call. Just sayin'. Abracadabra!

Heavenly Father,

Thank you for the physical care that I received from my wonderful doctors and also for the courage and hope their words infused into me. I'm so grateful. Please bless them. I pray now for all those going through health challenges. I pray that they have doctors who truly care and understand the power of the spoken word.

In Jesus' name, Amen.

FOR YOUR OWN READING: PSALM 30

32

Be Right or Be Happy

"Ego judges and punishes. Love
forgives and heals." ~Anonymous

ONCE HEARD THAT THE WORD *EGO* CAN STAND
for *Edging God Out.*

The older I get, the more I realize that when I get
wounded by a comment or when I feel left out or slighted, ten
times out of ten it's because my ego is governing the day. The
last thing in the world that I want to do is to edge God out.

The mechanism I've come to embrace at such times is
what I call the High Road. The High Road is simply a mental state in which I can get quiet. This mental state prevents
me from overanalyzing situations. It allows me to observe
what's happening at any given moment, and then, instead
of creating a story which can be a breeding ground for my
exaggerated sense of self-importance, I can understand that
in almost all cases, people are well-meaning and kind and
are trying to do the best they can. I will choose to believe

that they are not trying to hurt me. If, indeed, they are trying to hurt me, I can understand that it's probably not about me as I know that hurting people tend to hurt others.

Strangely enough, in most cases where I've chosen to take the High Road, the person involved seldom realizes it and probably never will. Therein lies my own personal growth.

Considering the fact that there have been a lot of times when I'd rather be right than happy, you can understand how this process is not always easy. My ego will occasionally fight to try and win the day. Yet, by God's grace, my ego loses the wrestling match with love every time.

Whether my choice to believe that people are well-meaning and trying to be kind is actually true or not, I've learned to get quiet with my thoughts, take a deep breath and say to myself, "It's all good!" Instead of edging God out, I can invite God in, pray about it and move my thoughts to a place of peace.

Like any other ego-driven human being, I have an innate way of collecting data to support whatever story I've created. If I want to collect data to support a story that someone is purposely trying to hurt me, believe me, I can find it. If I want to collect data to support my quest to take the High Road, believe me, I can find that as well. The first choice can lead to fear, self-absorption and an obsession for being right. The latter can lead to peace of mind and letting go. The first takes me back to a place that I've literally prayed myself out of. The latter takes me to a place that I've literally prayed myself into.

I've mentioned several times that I'm a verbal processor, so there are still times that I need to process out loud to a confidante – someone who knows that I don't need to be fixed. Someone who won't judge me during a struggle with my ego. Someone who allows me to listen to myself feeling sorry for myself, which, by the way, disgusts me. Someone who will pull me back to a place of self-esteem instead of self-importance.

Over the past several years, I've learned that everyone who is connected to me is not necessarily committed to me. There's a big difference, and I'm learning to recognize it. I'm truly okay with that. In fact, I'm grateful for it. It has allowed me to recognize the relationships that truly support my life and to let go of those relationships which can actually destroy what God has called me to do and be.

I've worked hard to stop saying to myself, "I can't believe how they're treating me." This has been a lengthy process and I've had to dig deep, but I've learned that the High Road is paved with productive and healthy questions. That's one of the reasons I like it there so much.

The High Road leads me to questions that aren't framed by feelings of entitlement or unexpressed expectations. Instead, I'm encouraged to ask questions that will result in an understanding that the world does not revolve around me. (Hard to believe, huh?) I can ask myself intelligent and thoughtful questions that will promote healing and peace instead of bitterness and division.

The questions are simple: How do I want to be treated? How do I want to treat others? (Golden Rule, anyone?) These questions flow from a state of quiet reflection and always remind me that I teach people how to treat me based on what I allow.

Afterwards, I'm able to decide whether to let something go or dig deeper with the one who has hurt, offended or slighted me. The High Road perspective helps me tremendously.

If I discover that I've allowed others to cross boundaries that I've set, I must ask myself if I've taken the time to communicate those boundaries to others. Once I've answered that question, it's my responsibility to decide if this person is one who values me and our relationship or someone whose relationship I can release with a silent blessing.

The alternative can be summed up with three R's: resentment, resistance and revenge. I resent how I'm treated. I begin to resist the one who hurt me. Then, subconsciously, I seek revenge by cutting that person out altogether. The devil uses these feelings to kill relationships and to mask hurts that can often be remedied if confronted with care.

At this stage of my life, when I'm hurt by someone, it's important for me to seek resolution immediately. Sometimes it takes a caring confrontation. Sometimes it's simply the process of asking myself the right questions to determine why I've allowed others to treat me in a manner inconsistent with the highest version of myself.

I'll ask myself, "What am I afraid of? Why don't I speak up?" When I mix these questions with my prayers for clarity, the air on the High Road always seems to clear.

I once read a quote that says, "*Somebody is discussing the old you because they don't have access to the new you.*"

I also heard a wise woman say, "*It's none of my business what other people think of me, and to tell you the truth, I really wouldn't care what they thought of me if I realized just how seldom they do.*" Serious truth right there.

When I travel the High Road I can remember that conflict won't survive when only one person participates. I can remember that feelings are just visitors unless we invite them to move in. After all, we *have* feelings, but we are *not* our feelings.

In the book of Matthew, Jesus was recorded as saying, "*Love the Lord your God with all your heart and with all your soul and with all your mind. And love your neighbor as yourself.*" This wasn't a suggestion; it was a command from the lips of God himself. I can't get around it, and there are no loopholes that I've discovered. It's non-negotiable.

I read the following quote recently: "*Love your neighbor even if they respond with ingratitude and contempt. All the more reason for the heroism of love. Would you be a featherbed warrior instead of bearing the rough fight of love? He who dares the most shall win the most; and if the path of love is rough, tread it boldly, still loving your neighbor through thick and thin. If they're hard to please, do not seek to please them, but to please your master; and remember if they spurn your love, your master has not spurned it, and your deed is as acceptable to him as if it had been acceptable to them. Love your neighbor, for in so doing you are following the footsteps of Christ."*

So, today and every day I will strive to travel the High Road. The traffic is light, the peace is profound, the communication is stellar, the vision is clear and love wins the day. Every time.

> Dear Heavenly Father,
> Help me to always travel the High Road in my relationships with others. With your help and guidance, I know that I can be a blessing to those who love me and help me. I thank you for your constant love and ask that your will is done in my life today.
> In Jesus' name, Amen.

FOR YOUR OWN READING: MATTHEW 22

33

Lean On Me

"You're safe not because of the absence of danger, but because of the presence of God." ~Unknown

I WAS DRIVING 70 MILES PER HOUR IN THE FAST lane of a freeway on a sunny afternoon in California. Traffic wasn't heavy, wasn't light. It was normal California traffic. I was on my way back to my mom's house after visiting my daughter and her family. Suddenly, from out of nowhere, I was rear ended by a hit-and-run driver who must have been going 90 miles per hour or more. At the time, I was on my hands-free phone talking to my daughter, and I didn't see this car coming up behind me. I found out later why I didn't see it coming, but I'll get to that in a minute.

The impact and terrible sound of that car hitting mine made me wonder if it was the end of the world. Sound dramatic? Well, for the record, a car hitting you from behind at that speed is dramatic and terrifying!

For a split second I didn't know what had happened, aside from the fact that my car was now being forced across all five lanes of the freeway. I started pumping the brakes, desperately trying to control my vehicle. Despite my best efforts, I totally lost control of the car.

I started yelling into the phone to my daughter, "Jorgi! Pray for me, pray for me, pray for me!" I don't know how many times I said that as I careened out of control across all five lanes of traffic.

She was yelling back, "Mama, mama, mama! Are you ok? Mama!" Then she began to yell to her three daughters, "Pray for Yia Yia! Pray for Yia Yia!"

My car continued up the embankment on the side of the freeway and proceeded to take out five trees. I had no idea where the trajectory of the vehicle would take me, but my hands gripped the wheel with a strength that I didn't know I had before the violence of the crash ripped them from the wheel.

I admit I don't actually recall if this happened, but in hindsight, I think Carrie Underwood's song *Jesus Take the Wheel* ran through my mind. What I do remember without a shadow of a doubt was that I felt everything slow down and thought to myself, "Is this how I'm going to die?" What a surreal and awful feeling. It was strange, even for me.

My good ol' car and I hit the fifth tree (yes, somehow I was counting them), and it finally stopped the car. The airbags deployed and I began to roll back down the embankment. Bystanders who witnessed the crash said I flipped five times. I finally landed upside down on the side of the freeway hanging from my seatbelt.

OnStar (God bless them!) immediately contacted me. The woman on the line calmly said, "This is OnStar; were you in an accident?" I had a quick vision of a movie scene where a car crashes and then blows up. The thought flashed through my mind at lightning speed.

I responded not so calmly, "Yes! And I'm hanging upside down and have to get out of this car!"

She calmly responded again, "An ambulance is on its way!"

I was still buckled in my seatbelt, hanging there, looking at the ceiling of my car, which now was below me. I knew I had to get out of my seat in order to drop onto the roof which was now the floor. Ugh. All of these thoughts were going through my mind when I realized that I was okay. I was okay! I think I thanked God, but to be honest, my dominant thought was, "I've got to get out of this car!"

With my thumb I pushed down on the red latch that kept my seatbelt secure, and immediately dropped onto the roof/floor of the car. I began to kick the window on the side of the car that I was on, trying desperately to get out.

It was then that I heard what I later called 'God with skin.' Many people who had been driving behind me had seen the erratic driver who hit me. Several of them had stopped when they saw what happened. They were talking and, although I didn't know what they were saying, the sound of their voices redirected my attention to the back of the car, instead of the window I was trying to kick out, which wasn't budging.

When I looked back at them, I saw that the back window had been completely blown out. All the glass was gone, and a group of people were standing outside the back of my car.

I saw my phone lying next to me. Although it had been disconnected from blue tooth during the crash, my daughter was still holding on, hearing everything going on. Ugh, and thank God!

I grabbed my phone and my purse and started crawling out of the car. As I was struggling to get out, I kept telling my daughter, "I'm ok. I'm crawling out! I'm crawling out!"

As I crawled out, I saw my youngest grandchild's car seat, on what was now the floorboard, which was the top of the car, torn from its regular place in the back seat. I crawled over or around it – I can't quite remember. My entire body was shaking with the thought that she could have been with me. I began to cry with thanksgiving! I used to say that fear and gratitude cannot dwell in the same mind, but in that moment, I promise you they did.

When I crawled out of the back window, there were two men, one young and on his phone to the police, another older guy and a young woman. As I stepped out of the car, all I can remember saying to her is, "Can you tell my daughter I'm okay?" With shaking hands I handed her my phone. Credit cards, license, yada, yada, all in this phone case, and I handed it to her like she was Mother Teresa. Maybe she was.

As she was talking to Jorgi, I said to her, "May I please lean on you for a moment?"

She said, "Of course!"

As I was leaning on her with my hand on her arm, I could hear her talking to Jorgi and reassuring her that I was okay.

My legs felt like rubber, so I attempted to sit down. My back hurt so much I couldn't do it. I kept trying to sit but would then stand back up with my back throbbing.

I should mention that as I stepped out of the car I saw a motorcycle policeman pulling up. In the midst of the chaos, he kindly started asking me questions. I can't remember all of them, but I do know he asked me for my name, date of birth and address, things I should quickly know. According to my daughter, I accurately gave him all the correct answers and she took a deep breath for the first time since I had been hit.

The older guy was standing next to me now. Still not being able to sit or stand very well, I said to him, "May I lean on you for a minute?"

He said, "Of course." This time, instead of taking his arm with my hand, I leaned on him as he put his arm around me for a moment. He said, "It's okay. It's okay."

By now, some other police cars had pulled up along with the paramedics and the fire department. I was asked a lot of questions and answered them with what I thought was a very clear, albeit frightened, mind.

My daughter was still on the phone with the young woman who said to me, "Do you want to just sit in my car and try to find some position that is more comfortable than standing or sitting while you answer these questions?" I took her up on her generous offer and found that leaning back in the seat helped me feel comfortable.

She asked Jorgi if she would like for her to take pictures of the car. Jorgi said, "Yes. Please!" The pictures of my wrecked car still send shivers down my spine as it seems impossible anybody could have survived the accident.

The next thing I knew, I was being put onto a gurney and into an ambulance with my phone and purse in hand.

The paramedics who arrived at the accident scene were unbelievable. They were calm, decisive, skilled. As I was put into the ambulance and pushed toward the front of it, I looked at the doors that would soon be closed near my feet. I knew I had been strapped in across my legs and, I think, somewhere on my upper body.

One of the paramedics was named Josh. I asked his name because I felt it was important to know the name of the man who had my life in his hands.

Josh calmly talked to me as he put an IV in my arm. I asked why he needed to do that. He calmly explained, "It's simply precautionary. Just in case you may need fluids or medication. This will expedite treatment at the hospital."

I said, "Do the windows on the back of this thing open?"

He said, "No, but I assure you, there is plenty of air in here! I'm right here, and I promise you, there's plenty of air. You're going to be fine."

I said, "Sorry. I can get a bit claustrophobic in closed spaces." Really, T?

He said, "No worries. Let me unstrap these." He unstrapped the belts across my legs.

I said, "Thank you, Josh, but why do my legs feel so heavy?"

He said, "Your purse is on them." He then lifted it off my legs. The heaviness on my legs left, and then I focused on my hands.

"Josh, my hands are buzzing. Is that normal?"

He said, "From what I can see, and from my experience, your hands are buzzing because you were just in a horrible car accident and your adrenaline is working overtime. That can cause your hands to buzz. Your blood pressure is fine, and we're on our way to the hospital now. We'll be there in no time."

I thought back to times in my life when my adrenaline was so ramped up that my hands started buzzing. The only thing that helped then was to take some deep cleansing breaths. So, that's what I did. I also began to recite the Lord's Prayer in my head. The buzzing stopped.

Josh asked me if I had any conditions he should know about.

I said, "No. Well, I do have a condition called situs inversus."

He said "You have what?"

I explained to him what it was. "It's a genetic condition where the organs in the chest and abdomen are positioned in a mirror image from their normal positions. For example, the left atrium of the heart and the left lung are positioned on the body's right side. In other words, all of my organs are switched."

He said, "Wow! Now that you mention it, I remember hearing about that when I was studying to be a paramedic, but I've never met anyone with it."

I said, "Well, there you go, Josh. I'm one in 10,000! Nice to meet you."

He laughed, and so did I.

To keep things light, I told him the story of when I found

out that my organs were switched. I was 16 when my mom changed us from our childhood pediatrician to a regular M.D. My mom and I were in an exam room with a new doctor and he was giving me a check-up. He checked my eyes, my nose, my mouth, my breathing. "Take a deep breath," he said. "Let it out." You know the drill. All was well. He came around to my front, placed his stethoscope on the left side of my chest and listened. His eyes grew wide. He listened again, and his eyes got wider. I looked at him, and my eyes grew wider as they mirrored his.

Unintentionally imitating Bugs Bunny, I said, "Nyahh, what's up, Doc?" I said, "Doc, lay it on the line! What's going on?"

He stepped back, looked at me, looked at my mom, then back at me and he said, "I can't hear your heart."

I said "What?"

Again he said, "I can't hear your heart."

I said, "Well, I'm breathing so I know it must be in there! Geez, man!"

He then listened for my heart on the right side of my chest and there it was, healthy and pounding away. He proceeded to tell me that I had a condition called dextrocardia. He assured us that it wasn't anything to worry about, but it was important for me to know. Ya think?

Once I was confident that it wasn't anything to be alarmed about, I proceeded to ask him if my boobs were in the back. I think this was an appropriate question considering how flat chested I was. He laughed. Good sign. I then said, "Hey, if they are in the back, I'd be fun for a guy to slow dance with, right?" Then he really laughed. So did my mom. So did I, and so did Josh as I was telling him the story in the back of an ambulance.

When I was 28, I had a dermoid cyst on my left ovary. It was benign, but it had to be removed. Prior to the surgery I had to have a barium enema. Ever had a barium enema? In the dictionary under *Are You Kidding Me?* it says, See *Barium Enema*. It was the worst!

Anyway, in the pictures from the enema they discovered that not only was my heart placement reversed, the rest of my organs were reversed as well. Good to know, people. Unbelievable.

I have to say, however, it was great material for my unexpected and unwanted ride to the hospital. My story gave Josh a good chuckle. As he was relaying need-to-know information to the nurse in the E.R., he couldn't tell her without laughing. It was a serious situation, but it was sense of humor for the win.

As much as I hated the scenario of the crash, I must tell you that the whole situation was filled with miracles. First of all, as horrible as it was for my daughter to be on the phone with me while it happened, I was able to request her to pray for me right then and there. In turn, she was able to yell to her daughters to pray for me right then and there. I know without a doubt and firmly believe that this called in my angels in a big way. There's no way I should have survived this crash except for the divine intervention of my guardian angels.

These Bible verses remain two of my favorites: *"For he will command his angels concerning you, to guard you in all your ways; they will lift you up in their hands, so that you will not strike your foot against a stone." Psalm 91:11-12* And *"The angel of the Lord encamps around those who fear him, and he delivers them." Psalm 34:7*

For years I have begun every day with this prayer: *"Thank you, God, that no evil shall befall me, my daughter or her family. No plague shall come near our dwellings. For you have sent our guardian angels to take charge over us and protect us. They keep us in all our ways. In our pathway is life, healing and health. In Jesus' name, Amen."*

I pray this prayer every morning and every night. The morning of the crash was no different.

There was a second miracle in play that day that I mentioned before. I'll expand on it now. While I was visiting my daughter and her family, I was looking at my youngest granddaughter, Elia, who was sitting on the couch across the room from me. This thought crossed my mind "Maybe I'll have her come and spend the night with me."

This was a normal thought for me when it comes to Elia. She was six years old at the time and we had had many sleepovers together. The only difference that day was the fact that I lived an hour from her instead of being only 15 minutes away.

As I considered asking to take her home that night, I thought to myself, "No, I don't know when I'll be able to get back down here, and I don't want the kids to have to come get her." So, without mentioning anything to her, I decided against it. Thank God!

As I crawled out of my totaled car, I saw her car seat in the back seat. I immediately knew that God had protected her and in doing so, protected me and our entire family because she wasn't with me during that crash. It was truly a miracle that God protected all of us that day.

The third miracle was that, due to how erratic the person was driving prior to hitting me, all of the cars on the freeway had backed away from us. Because he was in front of them, weaving all over the road, other drivers slowed down so that when I was forced across five lanes of the highway, not one single car hit me. On highway 80 in California, where everyone is going 70 to 80 miles an hour, this was without a doubt, a miraculous protection. God's protection for sure.

It's possible that some readers of this book will think of me surviving these events as nothing more than good luck. So be it. If you're not a person of faith, I can understand how you might think that. However, I'm 100% clear that I was not protected because of the absence of danger. I was protected because of the presence of God.

I also believe that if you understood the darkness from

which he delivered me, maybe then you will better understand the intensity of my worship, my devotion and my absolute clarity about these events.

As I was being dismissed from the trauma ward of the hospital, with a clear CT scan of my head and neck, a clear chest X-ray, a scratch on my arm, a couple small bruises on my legs and arms, a sore back and a bruised chest from the airbag, the doctor came into my room and said. "We've had a lot of people come in here whose cars looked like yours. Trust me when I tell you, they didn't look like you."

I said, "I'm clear how blessed I am. And, for that, I praise Jesus! Thank you for taking care of me. God bless you."

She said, "Yes. And thank you."

I walked out of the emergency room. No wheelchair. Nobody escorting me. I walked out straight into the arms of my daughter and my eldest granddaughter who, due to Covid, had been waiting for me outside the E.R. My daughter looked at me and said, "I cannot believe that you just walked out of there!"

I said, "I know. It's all God. It was my angels. It was prayer. It was divine protection. I am so grateful. I am so blessed."

Together they said, "Yes!"

We held each other and cried. Finally, we got in the car and drove back to their house, where I would stay for a few days to rest and recover.

The day I needed to return to my mom's, my daughter asked me if I'd like for her to drive me. I told her that as nervous as I was to drive again, especially on the same highway where it all happened, I had to do it. I had made the decision that I wouldn't allow the experience, or the fear that it created, to control me. After all, the way I saw it then and still see it now, is the greatest risk I'll ever take is not taking one.

I've reflected quite often on the crash itself. I still think about it each time I get in my car to drive somewhere. Facing that initial fear is something I had to do and something that I still have to overcome in order to live the life I want to live.

I pray for God to lessen the memory of the crash itself. Instead, I ask him to magnify the miracles in my mind. I thank him over and over again for his protection and for his grace.

I'm very aware that the dark side wants me to worry about my future so I can't enjoy my life right now. I'm also aware that the devil is a liar and the father of lies, so I am determined to enjoy every minute of my life because each day is a gift from God. *"The Lord himself goes before you and is with you. He will never leave you nor forsake you. Do not be afraid; do not be discouraged." Deuteronomy 31:8*

I'll never know (this side of heaven) why I was able to walk away from such a terrible accident when others in the same situation might have been crippled or killed. I don't take this lightly. At all! Yet, I don't ask God why, because, in my experience, he doesn't always answer why. I know and understand that his ways are not always our ways.

I do thank him and my angels over and over. I ask him what he still wants me to do, as I know he saved me that day.

My friend Kathy personalized this scripture promise for me after I went through my second round of chemotherapy and radiation treatments. I've had it pasted to my bathroom mirror ever since.

"I will instruct you, Thea, and guide you, Thea, in the way you should go. I will watch over you, Thea, and counsel you, Thea, says the Lord." ~Psalm 32:8

I read it daily and take it for the promise that it is. I've always understood how important it is to pray, but after the accident, I've learned that it's just as important to praise.

I've learned to lean on God's provision, but more importantly, to worship him as the provider.

Finally, I've learned that *"At the name of Jesus, every knee will bow, of those who are in heaven and on earth and under the earth!" Philippians 2:10* And *"If we don't praise our Lord, the rocks themselves will cry out their praises." Luke 19:39-40*

As for the man who hit me, I can't even begin to fathom

the darkness that must be surrounding his soul in order for him to have made the choices he made that day. It's unimaginable.

He took the first exit off the freeway, parked his car and fled. I pray that they catch him, so he can't ever do this again. Yet, at the time of this writing, the authorities know who he is but have been unable to find him.

There's a saying, "You can run, but you cannot hide." A better rendition is Biblical: *"If I go up to the heavens, you are there; if I make my bed in the depths, you are there." Psalm 139:8*

Yep. God knows the identity of the man who hit me and then ran. God knows where he is. In the end, I leave it in his hands.

I have at times prayed for this man and for his soul. More importantly, I've forgiven him. I've forgiven him because the question isn't "How much forgiveness does he deserve?" The question is "How much peace and freedom do I desire?" Forgiveness doesn't excuse his behavior. Forgiveness prevents his behavior from destroying my heart.

Finally, as I look back on this experience, I realize how it changed me and how it shaped me. It's given me empathy for those who have fears I may not have, and it has called me deeper into the Word and the beauty of all God's promises. It has deepened my faith and helped me to lean on God more than ever before. He is always there for me.

"Yet you, Lord, are our Father. We are the clay, you are our potter; we are all the work of your hand." ~Isaiah 64:8

To him be the glory, forever and ever.

Dear Lord,

Thank you for your divine protection in our lives. The times we know about and the times we don't. Thank you for our guardian angels who continuously watch over us and protect us. "Lord, you have examined me and know all about me. You know when I sit down and when I get up. You know my thoughts before I think them. You know where I go and where I lie down. You know everything I do. Lord even before I say a word, you already know it. You are all around me – in front and in back – and have put your hand on me. Your knowledge is amazing to me; it is more than I can understand." Psalm 139:1 – 6

In Jesus' precious name, Amen.

FOR YOUR OWN READING: PSALM 139

34
Doubt Your Doubts

"A heart full of faith is better
than a soul full of doubts."
~Matshona Dhliwayo

T HIS MIGHT SOUND TERRIBLE, BUT I WAS HAPPY
to read that at one point in his life, the late Rev. Billy
Graham struggled with his faith. I'd read about this years
ago in one of his books and was reminded of it recently after
reading an article written by Will Graham, his grandson.

He wrote, "While my grandfather had always accepted in
his head the authority of the Scriptures, there was a turning
point in which a very good friend of his, a man named Charles
Templeton, had begun challenging his way of thinking."

Mr. Templeton, who had preached with Youth for Christ
as well, had gone on to study at Princeton, where he started
to believe that the Bible was flawed and that academia, not
Jesus, was the answer to life's problems and that the Bible
couldn't be trusted.

Billy Graham began to wonder if he even believed the very book from which he was preaching. Should he follow Templeton in questioning its validity?

Ultimately, he was invited by a well-known and godly woman named Henrietta Mears to preach at Forest Home, a Christian retreat. Henrietta took some grief for inviting Graham to preach because he was not part of the camp's denomination, but God had a plan.

The article goes on to say that Billy Graham struggled with the Lord. Billy Graham? Struggled with the Lord? Hard to comprehend.

However, while at Forest Home, Billy Graham had an experience that would profoundly change the course of his ministry and affect the eternal address of millions of people.

Rev. Graham walked out into the woods one day and set his Bible on a tree stump and cried out, "Oh, God! There are many things in this book I do not understand. There are many problems with it for which I have no solution. There are many seeming contradictions. There are some areas in it that do not seem to correlate with modern science. I can't answer some of the philosophical and psychological questions that Chuck and others are raising."

Then Billy Graham fell to his knees and the Holy Spirit moved in him as he said, "Father, I am going to accept this as your Word by faith! I'm going to allow faith to go beyond my intellectual questions and doubts, and I will believe this to be your inspired Word."

He never looked back. Because of that tree stump moment of decision and complete faith, millions of people have learned about Jesus Christ as their Lord and Savior and will spend eternity with him.

The rest of the story is rather sad. In 1957, Charles Templeton publicly declared that he had become an agnostic.

Some fifty years later, Lee Strobel had an opportunity to interview Templeton, who had just a couple more years to live. He was in his 80s and was suffering from Alzheimer's but was still a clear conversation partner. In *A Case for Faith*, Strobel recounts the ending of their wide-ranging conversation.

"And how do you asses this Jesus?" he asked Templeton. It seemed like the next logical question, but he wasn't prepared for the response it would evoke.

Strobel wrote, "Templeton's body language softened. It was as if he suddenly felt relaxed and comfortable in talking about an old and dear friend. His voice, which at times had displayed such a sharp and insistent edge, now took on a melancholy and reflective tone. His guard seemingly down, he spoke in an unhurried pace, almost nostalgically, carefully choosing his words as he talked about Jesus."

"He was," Templeton began, "the greatest human being who has ever lived. He was a moral genius. His ethical sense

210

was unique. He was the intrinsically wisest person that I've ever encountered in my life or in my readings. His commitment was total and led to his own death, much to the detriment of the world. What could one say about him except that this was a form of greatness?"

Strobel was taken aback. "You sound like you really care about him," he said.

"Well, yes. He is the most important thing in my life," came his reply. He stuttered, searching for the right words, "I...I...I know it may sound strange, but I have to say...I adore him."

"Everything good I know, everything decent I know, everything pure I know, I learned from Jesus. Yes! Yes! And tough? Just look at Jesus. He castigated people. He got angry. People don't think of him that way, but they don't read the Bible. He had a righteous anger. He cared for the oppressed and the exploited. There's no question that he had the highest moral standard, the least duplicity, the greatest compassion of any human being in history. There have been many other wonderful people, but Jesus is Jesus!"

"But, no," he said slowly. "He's the most..." He stopped and then started again. "In my view," Templeton declared, "he is the most important human being who has ever existed. And if I may put it this way," he said as his voice began to crack, "I...miss...him!"

With that, tears flooded his eyes. He turned his head and looked downward, raising his left hand to shield his face from Strobel. His shoulders bobbed as he wept.

Templeton fought to compose himself. Strobel could tell that it wasn't like him to lose his composure in front of a stranger. He sighed deeply and wiped away a tear. After a few more awkward moments, he waved his hand dismissively. Finally, quietly but adamantly, he said, "Enough of that."

Based on this conversation with Lee Strobel, I have no doubt that Mr. Templeton was a beautiful human being. Still, it strikes me as incredibly sad that, while Billy Graham, in his tree stump moment chose faith in Jesus and understood his Word to be truth, Charles Templeton allowed his intellect to create such doubt that he could not believe.

I know people like that. People who do not believe that the Bible is the true Word of God. People who believe that Jesus was a great man, a great teacher, a prophet. But they don't believe that he is the Son of God. I don't know the Bible by heart. I don't have the intellect of Charles Templeton or even of some friends of mine who doubt. What I have is faith. Pure and simple. I have a firm knowing in my spirit that Jesus is the Son of the Living God. That he was both God and man at the same time. That he loves all mankind.

To be honest, I'm glad I'm not an intellectual. *"For it is written: 'I will destroy the wisdom of the wise; the intelligence of the intelligent I will frustrate.'" 1 Corinthians 1:19*

From the moment I heard about Billy Graham's decision to doubt his doubts and to allow God to use him, I did the same thing. Never for a single moment would I compare myself to Billy Graham. I am, however, comparing his decision to doubt his doubts and to believe without pause to the choices I have made.

I'm clear that my faith rests solely on the fact that Jesus Christ is the Son of God and that he is my only way to heaven. I recognize that this is not a popular view in a lot of circles these days. I've been accused of having 'head-in-the-sand' faith, and that's okay. The Holy Spirit comes where he is loved, where he is invited, where he is expected. For those who don't believe, I can understand how challenging it might be to understand my faith.

One of the reasons I wrote this book was to share my faith with others. There are three businesses. My business, your business and God's business. All I can do is plant seeds of faith in my fellow human beings, pray for them and then let the Holy Spirit do his work.

He was there at the tree stump moment for Billy Graham. He was there with me in a small chapel in Mt. Hermon, California, when I stood alone at 16 years of age and gave my heart and life to Jesus Christ. I've failed. I've strayed. I've lived according to my own selfish will. By the grace of God, however, I have never lost my faith. I pray that this gift will strengthen me the rest of my life, so that I can dwell in the house of the Lord forever!

Heavenly Father,

Thank you for giants of faith who have gone before me. Thank you for my faith in Jesus. Only because of that can I know you and your infinite love for me and all sinners. Bless me this day as I share my faith with others.

In Jesus' name, Amen.

FOR YOUR OWN READING: 1 CORINTHIANS 1

35
Humble Pie

"True humility is not thinking less of yourself; it is thinking of yourself less." ~Rick Warren

W HEN YOU THINK YOU'RE THE SMARTEST ONE in the room, it might be time to find a new room.

At the point in my career when I had been in business for 27 years, I naturally assumed that I was proficient, skilled, and had most, if not all, the answers when it came to building people. I naturally assumed that I could climb the next rung on the ladder of success with ease. I was completely wrong in both my assumptions.

The one thing I learned, more than any other thing that I've discovered about advancement, is that I had to humble myself to the following idea: people in other rooms knew more than me, and I needed them. Not only that, but I had to acknowledge that I needed them. I had to get off my high horse and seek their counsel. I had to change the thought that since I had been with our company as long as or longer than others, I was above learning from them. Yes, I had read a zillion books on leadership. I had practiced my skills for years. Still, I could learn from others and absorb knowledge from those in the position I aspired to achieve.

Knowledge has little to do with longevity. Longevity has more to do with desire and the willingness, even humility, to keep learning. I had to become hungry enough for the next level that I could put aside all my status-quo knowledge and humbly ask for help.

I found a new room. A room where I was uncomfortable. A room where I could admit that what I had been doing, although successful in the eyes of many who were not striving for a similar goal, was not going to get me where I wanted to be.

Well, guess what? That new room was filled with women who had gone before me, who had done the same things that I had done. They accepted my newfound humility and honored me in it. They shared. They cared. They listened. They coached. They supported. No matter how it looked from the outside, they were completely different than I was prior to entering the room.

I am forever grateful that I entered that room. Thank God! It not only changed my position and the security of my future, but it changed my rolodex, my circle of friends and the trajectory of my life.

I have found that it's easier for most people to stay stuck in their own sense of assuming they know everything. Been there, done that. If you are in a room where you feel like you are the smartest person there, even though you haven't gotten to where you'd like to be, it might be time to find a new room.

Heavenly Father,

I thank you for putting people in my life that helped me grow. You have gifted me with many talents and abilities, and I'm grateful that you put people in my life that helped me use them and expand them. I ask today that you would continue to help me be a blessing to others as they strive to be all that you created them to be.

In Jesus' name, Amen.

FOR YOUR OWN READING: PROVERBS 11

36
Run to Him

"Very early in the morning, while
it was still dark, Jesus got up, left
the house and went off to a solitary
place, where he prayed." ~Mark 1:35

AS MUCH AS I'VE TRIED TO AVOID IT, I WOULD
be remiss if I didn't speak of the Covid-19 pandemic.
To be honest, the reason I feel compelled to write about
it has little to do with the pandemic itself. Rather, it's more
about how I've come to realize what happened to my soul in
the midst of it.

I feel as though my soul has been tested more during the
past two years than ever before. My soul, my mind, my will
and my emotions. As much as I don't care to dwell on it,
if I don't remain acutely aware of what's going on around
me in the world, and without an intentional resolve to keep
my joy, the isolation and fear caused by this pandemic often
becomes stifling and claustrophobic.

Like many others, I've grown tired and weary, (there's a difference) even scared sometimes, wondering if it will ever end. It seems to be the focus of every conversation, the root of many disagreements and the center of great conflict between people, even believers. At times, it's like a colorless and odorless gas, spreading darkness and fear. It can be all encompassing.

I woke up recently with an all-too-familiar feeling of anxiety. I had a lot on my mind. I had concerns that had turned to worry, and it felt like I was suffocating. I began to pray, yet the weight of the feelings grew heavier. I felt a sense of foreboding that seemed to reach deep into my heart and soul. Once again, I thought to myself, "How can I have such faith and still feel such fear?"

I got out of bed, opened the shutters to allow the light of the day to settle into my home, gave Eddie some fresh water and made a hot cup of coffee. I grabbed my Bible and my current devotional, went into the backyard, sat myself down and began to get into God's Word.

Immediately, my feelings of darkness and fear began to disappear. I became aware of an overwhelming sense of awe and appreciation. The Holy Spirit was ministering to my soul.

The words that I read spoke peace and blessings to the same heart that, just 20 minutes earlier, had been gripped with anxiety. As I continued to read and to pray, the anxiety slowly melted away and peace began to take its place.

I began to pray. I cried out to my heavenly Father, and he answered me in my spirit.

"Thea, although this has been your routine for many years, little by little you have allowed the state of the world and the all-consuming conversations about the state of the world, along with your current responsibilities, to overrun your thought life. Because of that, you have only fit me in whenever you couldn't take it anymore. I am no longer your priority. For several months, you have been missing an important part of your routine. This change has radically changed you, your feelings of peace, your faith and your perception of life."

As I continued to pray, it dawned on me what I had been leaving out: priority and praise. Yes, priority and praise!

Before the world was turned upside down by Covid-19, I would open the window coverings no matter where I lived and the very first words I would say out loud were, "Good morning, God! I love you, God! Great is your faithfulness!"

I said this every single morning after I woke up. It got to the point that when I'd spend the night with my youngest granddaughter, when we'd wake up, I'd open the blinds and she would instantly say, "Good morning, God! I love you, God!" Priority and praise was our routine.

Only then would I continue the rest of my routine. Open the shutters, get my coffee, my Bible and my devotional. I'd fill my mind and soul with the Word of God and praise him again for his faithfulness. I'd ask him to forgive my sins and then pray for my family and friends. Then I'd talk to him about my concerns and my responsibilities and ask him to guide me in thought, word and deed.

I promise you, I would never pretend to be holier than you. This was just my daily routine that helped me survive. It was the only way I knew how to function above all the worries that tried to keep me from spending time with God. Your routine will undoubtedly be different but just as effective.

I once read that Satan doesn't try to rob an empty house. How true! Sadly, during this strange time in our world, I've allowed him to remain a thief in my soul for far too long.

No wonder there were days when I'd wake up feeling anxious and fearful. How could my soul be at peace when it wasn't in praise? How could my spirit find joy when I was just fitting God in?

I was wearing out from being weary. All of this had been going on as I wrote this book. Amazing, no? Yet, until I got quiet in my backyard prayer room, I didn't fully understand that even though I was talking and writing about God nearly every day, I was still just fitting him in.

Another relevant thought came to me as I wrote this chapter. How would I feel as a mom if my beautiful child just fit me in and only wanted me around to get something from me? How would I feel if she never expressed appreciation? Not so good, I'm sure.

Ultimately, instead of going to God, the Creator of the universe, the Alpha and Omega, the Everlasting to Everlasting, I would text a friend and try to explain what was going on. I'd ask her to pray for me, all the while forgetting that she was *not* the Creator of the universe, the Alpha and Omega, the Everlasting to Everlasting.

I probably shouldn't be surprised by this, but I never paid attention to the fact that I never left one of those conversations, whether text or voice, feeling the peace that passes all understanding. Not once. Until I wrote this and pondered it, I wasn't even aware of how far off course I had gotten.

If Jesus needed to go to a solitary place to spend time with his Father alone, to pray, what made me think I could possibly live the life that he died to give me, or fulfill his calling for my life without doing the same?

You might be thinking, "It's easy for you to have a routine like this. You're retired. You don't live my life. You don't have my schedule or my demands. You don't have to get a family up and off to school or get ready for a busy day at work." I get that. 100%.

I would never judge how you spend time with God, nor would I ever tell you how to live out your faith. I'm sharing this only because this is what has worked for me.

Let me finish by saying that I have followed a variance of this routine throughout many seasons in my life. It was different when I was single, when I went through a divorce, when I was a single mom, when I met and married Lyle and when I was raising my daughter from infancy to empty nest.

My prayer closet was different during each season as well. Sometimes it would be in my shower, where I couldn't read the Word but could still pray and praise. Sometimes it was in an actual prayer room in my home where I could luxuriate in the time that I was able to spend with God. Sometimes, my prayer room was nature itself. I would pray as I walked outside. My current routine is wonderful because I have more free time to spend with God. The praying and praising has never really changed.

The seasons of my life were all very different, but I always found time to spend with God, who never changes! *"He is the same yesterday, today and tomorrow." Hebrews 13:8*

Yep. While writing this, I realized that my routine had changed. Because of that, I had changed. Thank God that he is relentless in his love for me and his desire is for me to remain close to him. His love and faithfulness are boundless. Only by his mercy can I return to my routine of putting him first in prayer and praise instead of just fitting him in when I'm anxious and worried.

I love it when he says to me, "Welcome back, my child!"

Dear Father,

It's not the time of day but the time itself that I spend with you that refreshes my soul. Keep me mindful of my need for you. Thank you for your incomprehensible love, and for the way you pursue me when I stray. Help me to know, that although I do not know what the future holds, you hold the future. You know the end at the beginning. You have redeemed me and nothing I do can separate me from your love.

In Jesus' name, Amen.

FOR YOUR OWN READING: HEBREWS 13

This world is not your home
and yet I am with you,
So, run to me my child, run to me.
My arms are open wide and my love
for you is infinite, so, run to me.
Run to me and I will always catch you.
Let me hold you in my arms and
whisper in your ear that I love you.
Run to me.
I will lift you up, like a loving
father would lift their child.
Run to me.
You are mine. I call you by name.
~Thea Elvin

37

Youth is a Gift, Age is an Art

"In the end, it's not the years in your life that count, it's the life in your years." ~Abraham Lincoln

WHEN I WAS MOVING INTO MY NEW HOME, I started to pack up my mom's things a few pieces at a time. One day I opened a drawer in a side table in the living room. The house where we were staying was over 50 years old. In those days, most houses were built with living rooms instead of family rooms. When I went to stay with my mom, no one was hanging out there anymore, so the drawers hadn't been touched for a long time.

Inside this particular drawer were a bunch of table coasters. One of them caught my attention. On it was inscribed, "Youth is a gift. Age is an art." It reminded me of a line from

It's a Wonderful Life, one of my all-time favorite movies. "Ah! Youth! It's wasted on the young!"

I don't know what Philip Van Doren Stern meant when he wrote that line, but I know there have been plenty of times in my life when I didn't appreciate my family, my home, my friends, my education, my church, my faith or my health the way I do now. I know I took these things for granted when I was young. Today I cherish these same things with every fiber of my being.

If age is an art, think about this. If you live to be into your 90's, it's as if things return to when you were a baby. When you were born, you didn't have much hair, you couldn't hear well, you couldn't walk, couldn't talk, could barely see. You drooled, needed diapers, and had to be cared for 24 hours a day. If you live long enough, you'll relive many of the same things.

My maternal grandmother lived to be 104 years old. She was blind in one eye and could barely see out of the other. She couldn't hear worth a darn and couldn't walk without a walker. I don't know if she lived her last days in the convalescent home in diapers, but I would imagine she did. She was cared for and watched over 24 hours a day.

It's true. Youth is wasted on the young. It's there, and then, in what seems to be a second, it's gone. The trippy thing about it is that when you're in it, you don't even realize it, yet alone appreciate it. Life just flows on by. As a kid you experience both good and bad; all your experiences are melded into what will become your life down the road.

The night I cleaned out that drawer was a beautiful night where I was living at the time. I'd watched some TV with my mom and was getting ready for bed. I had let Eddie out into the backyard and sat down to wait for him to do his business. I looked up into the sky. The night was warm and the sky was clear. There was a beautiful quarter moon that looked as if God had hung it in the sky just for me. The stars were twinkling. I prayed, "God, You not only created the stars, you know each of them by name."

I thought about the only thing I had been a part of creating: my daughter, Jorgi. She had called me that night a couple of hours before as she drove home from work. She told me about her day. We talked about the kids and her plans for her day off. It was lovely and I cherished every second of our call.

I missed my daughter with an overwhelming ache that represented all the love and admiration I felt for her. As she talked about her daughters, my memories of her childhood bubbled up in my heart. I realized more than ever that her youth was a gift – one that went by way too quickly. For both of us, no doubt.

At the same time, I felt this overwhelming feeling that my age had truly become a gift. I know so much more than I did in my youth. I appreciate things more than ever. Things that I overlooked in my youth. When I saw the words on the coaster at my mom's house, the phrase 'age is an art' felt like my personal truth.

I felt joy in every reflection. I thought, she is no longer a child, yet I was able to live in her life during her youth. It was a gift to her, but more importantly, it was a gift for me.

Youth is a gift; age is an art. Now she's passing on her many lessons to her three daughters who are in their youth. They probably don't appreciate it yet, but someday they will.

My child has now become my friend. I respect her more than I can express. I have so much pride in her and so much gratitude for her.

Age is an art when memories fill your heart, but you learn to live in the present.

Age is an art when your past unfolds as lessons for your future, as well as the futures of your children. Age is an art when you can embrace each passing year with joy.

Heavenly Father,
Thank you for life. For love. For family. Thank you for your perfect plan amidst the changes and challenges, joys and heartaches. Thank you for the

memories of the past and hopes for the future for generations to come. May they live life as an art, as they age, even when they don't know it.

In Jesus' name, Amen.

FOR YOUR OWN READING: 1 TIMOTHY 4

38

For You

"The weight that lies on your
shoulders could be the wings that
carry you home." ~Anonymous

A T THIS POINT IN MY LIFE AND DURING THIS
period of my new found love of writing, I have no idea
if anybody will read what I've written. That, my friends,
is in God's hands.

If you've picked up this book and read this far, I'd like to
address those of you who are hurting. I want you to know
that you are not alone. I'd like to remind you of some special
words that Jesus himself said: *"I have told you these things,
so that in me you may have peace. In this world you will have
trouble. But take heart! I have overcome the world." John 16:33*

God is with you. You may not feel him at times. There
are times when I don't feel him. If you're going through
something that seems unbearable, hang on. His love for
you isn't contingent upon your understanding of his ways. I

personally believe that even by questioning God's presence, at least you are talking to him.

If you're like me, you probably have many questions for him. Perhaps that is why the Word gives us a heads up on all of our challenges.

This Bible verse has sustained me, challenged me and blessed me throughout my adult life: *"For my thoughts are not your thoughts, neither are your ways my ways," declares the Lord. "As the heavens are higher than the earth, so are my ways higher than your ways and my thoughts than your thoughts."*

With that I can say, "I won't question God's will for my life."

You might ask, "Why?"

The answer is simple. Many questions that you and I have won't be answered this side of heaven.

As I put the finishing touches on this book, my heartfelt prayer was that each reader would understand that, although I've experienced heartbreak, fear, loneliness, sorrow and sadness, the one constant through it all has been my faith in the God of the universe.

His love for me has been evident every day of my life, even when I was so sad that I couldn't feel it at certain times. His faithfulness continues to lift my spirits.

He has loved me when I failed, lifted me out of my pits of

despair, restored my joy, my vision and my empathy. I pray that in some way, my story will help you or anybody else who has lived in the dark. I pray that my life experiences will help reveal to you the light of God's great love. I pray that his promises will illuminate your mind and bolster your soul.

Looking back on my life there are many things I would do differently if given the chance. Yet, when I put it all together, even things that I wish I could change were used for good and for God's purpose in my life. *"Therefore, brothers and sisters, I do not consider myself yet to have taken hold of it. Forgetting what is behind and straining toward what is ahead, I press on toward the goal to win the prize for which God has called me heavenward in Christ Jesus." Philippians 3:13-14*

I will continue to hold on to his promises, knowing that the answers to all my questions are wrapped firmly in his unending love for me. *"For I know the plans I have for you,"* declares the Lord, *"plans to prosper you and not to harm you, plans to give you a hope and a future." Jeremiah 29:11*

Gracious Heavenly Father,

Thank you for loving me each day. Thank you for providing direction and guidance in my life. Even though I don't always understand your will for my life, I hold on to your promises and trust that you always have my best interests at heart. Help me line up today with your will so that I can follow your commands and be a good example for others.

In Jesus' name, Amen.

FOR YOUR OWN READING: JOHN 3

39
Your Body Hears Everything Your Mind Says

"You never know what you can do until you try, and very few try unless they have to." ~C.S. Lewis

AS I CAME TO THE END OF THIS MANUSCRIPT, I wanted to add some final comments about how important your self-talk can be. For me, it seems to be the only thing that I can actually control. My body hears everything my mind says. Every single thing.

There's a scene in Mel Gibson's *Passion of the Christ* where Jesus (played by Jim Caviezel) is carrying his own cross to Golgotha, the place of his crucifixion. He stumbles and falls several times, and finally, the cross lands on top of him. Guards were whipping him; people were yelling at him.

His mother, who was in the crowd, runs to him. While she's running, she has a flashback to when Jesus was a little boy and had fallen and hurt himself. She ran to him then too, picked him up and cradled him in her arms. The mother of Jesus cradled God in her arms.

This time, as Jesus lay underneath the burden of his own cross, she could not pick him up or cradle him. She could only weep.

Jesus looked up at his mother and said, "See, Mother, behold, I make all things new."

Regardless of the place in the Bible from which Gibson took that passage, it doesn't really matter. That's exactly what Jesus did on the cross – he made all things new.

"*My body hears everything my mind says,*" is such a simple quote, but sometimes the simple ones are the most profound. This quote hit me so hard that I immediately wrote it on my bathroom mirror so I'd be reminded of it every day.

I've learned to survive life's hits while still being able to cherish life's blessings. How? By falling back on my faith and leaning into the wonderful promises of God that fill his holy Word.

From the day of his birth to his eventual death and resurrection, Jesus made all things new. Today, in our upside down world filled with sadness and disappointments, blessings and beauty, Jesus continues to make all things new. "*But*

God demonstrates his own love for us in this: while we were still sinners, Christ died for us."

Dearest Jesus,

Thank you for making all things new. Thank you for the promise of eternal life which is mine as a result of your sacrifice. Bless me this day and help me keep my eyes fixed on you.

In Jesus' name, Amen.

FOR YOUR OWN READING: MATTHEW 22

40
What's in a Name?

"The story is truly finished and meaning is made, not when the author adds the last period, but when the reader enters." ~Celeste Ng

MY DAD WAS SMART. NOT JUST COMMONSENSE smart but educated smart.

One day I asked him, "Pop, what was the greatest academic lesson you ever learned in college?"

Without skipping a beat he said, "I was in an English class, and we were assigned a book to read. We were told that we would be tested on it the following week. I read the entire book and felt ready for the exam. When it came time to take the exam, our instructor handed it to us and told us that we had the entire class period to complete it. I looked at the paper and there was only one question on it: 'Who was the author?' I failed the exam. From that day on, I never read anything without knowing who wrote it."

From my dad's lesson, I've tried to do the same.

As I struggled with the ups and downs of writing this book, I've come to appreciate the lesson that professor was teaching his students. Writing is hard work requiring great discipline. To author a book takes commitment, faith, grit, and in my case, tremendous grace. I nearly gave up on it many times. Comparing myself to authors whose writing I respect and admire was a humbling exercise. All too often, a voice (sometimes loud) in my head would tell me that I wasn't up to the task or that nobody would appreciate my work, yet I persisted.

My name is Thea Elvin, and I wrote this book.

Dear Heavenly Father,

Thank you for leading me through the process of writing this book. I couldn't have done it without you. I pray that my words will be a blessing to others, and as I have prayed throughout the process, "May the words of my mouth, and the mediation of my heart, be acceptable in Thy sight, O Lord, my strength, and my redeemer."

In Jesus' precious name, Amen and Amen.

FOR YOUR OWN READING: COLOSSIANS 1

Acknowledgements

T O MY DEAR FRIENDS AND FAMILY MEMBERS who listened to a chapter or two as I was putting words to the page: The time you took to listen and your cherished words of encouragement kept me going when it would have been easier to quit. May God put an extra jewel in each of your crowns for your belief in me and for your help. Thank you. I love you.

To Jan Karon, Max Lucado, Suzie Larson, Anne Graham-Lotz and Francine Rivers: Your work makes me want to write, and your work makes me afraid to write. As I stepped out of my comfort zone to write this book, I tried not to compare myself to you on any level. Even though you don't know me, you inspired me to continue working throughout the process. Your great talent for writing helped me aspire to be better in everything I do. Your words have forever blessed my life. May you all live to be 100 years old with pen still in hand, changing the world for Christ! Thank you.

To Dan Madson, my gifted editor and publisher: Thank you for never negotiating with my doubts or my fears regarding the manifestation of this book. Your devotion to detail and excellence is evident in all you do. This project was no exception. Thank you for the countless hours you spent teaching me to be a better writer, all the while encouraging me to continue. The editing process takes skill, brains and heart – along with understanding and caring about the author's intended message. The tears we shed as we worked together gave me the confidence to trust myself as I put my thoughts down on the page. Your devotion was love in action. You have honored Lyle after his death, as you did during his life. In doing so you have honored me and all who love him. Not only that, but you are the grandfather to my grandchildren, and I love you for that. You are a gift. May God continue to shower you with his grace and blessings.

To Liz Nitardy, my talented cover designer: Your love of Jesus is reflected in the way you live and the way you give. I'm incredibly fortunate that you have used your talents to create the cover for this book. It's a work of art and reveals the contents within so beautifully. I can't thank you enough, Liz. God bless you.

To Lyle. I will miss you every day of my life. Thank you for loving me.

To Jesus, my Savior: *"For God so loved the world, that he gave his only begotten Son, that whosoever believes in him should not perish, but have everlasting life." ~John 3:16* Thank you. I love you.

About the Author

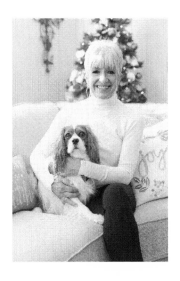

THEA ELVIN IS A RETIRED MARY KAY Independent National Sales Director. She lives in north-ern California where she cares for her aging mom and enjoys spending time with Eddie, her Cavalier King Charles Spaniel. When she's not educating, coaching and mentoring other businesswomen around the country, Thea loves to travel, cook, read, write and spend time with her daughter and son-in-law, granddaughters, family and friends.

Notes

_____
_____
_____
_____
_____
_____
_____
_____
_____
_____
_____
_____
_____
_____
_____
_____
_____
_____
_____

_____
_____
_____
_____
_____
_____
_____
_____
_____
_____
_____
_____
_____
_____
_____
_____
_____
_____
_____
_____
_____
_____
_____
_____